An Atlas of Normal Skeletal Scintigraphy

An Atlas of Normal Skeletal Scintigraphy

James J. Flanagan
MB FFR
Consultant Radiologist
Pembury Hospital and
Tunbridge Wells District

Michael N. Maisey
MD FRCP FRCR
Consultant Physician
and Head of Department of Nuclear Medicine
Guy's Hospital, London

Wolfe Medical Publications Ltd

Copyright © James J. Flanagan, Michael N. Maisey, 1985
Published by Wolfe Medical Publications Ltd, 1985
Printed by Butler & Tanner Ltd, Frome, England
ISBN 07234 0829 7

For a full list of titles published by Wolfe Medical Publications Ltd please write to the publishers at: Wolfe House, 3 Conway Street, London W1P 6HE, England

All rights reserved. The contents of this book, both photographic and textual, may not be reproduced in any form, by print, photoprint, phototransparency, microfilm, microfiche, or any other means, nor may it be included in any computer retrieval system, without written permission from the publishers.

Contents

Preface	7	Anterior view of thoracic cage	38
Anterior view of whole body	8	Posterior view of thoracic cage	40
Posterior view of whole body	9	Posterior view of thoracic spine	42
Anterior view of skull	10	Oblique lumbar spine	44
Lateral skull	12	Posterior view of lumbar spine	46
Turned oblique view of cervical spine	14	Anterior view of pelvis	48
Posterior view of cervical spine	16	Posterior view of pelvis	50
Anterior view of clavicle	18	Sacro-iliac joints	52
Anterior view of left shoulder	20	Posterior view of sacrum	54
Posterior view of scapula	22	Posterior view of hip	56
Anterior view of left humerus	24	Anterior view of femur	58
Anterior view of elbow joint	26	Lateral view of knee	60
Lateral view of elbow	28	Posterior view of knee	62
Anterior view of forearm	30	Anterior view of tibia and fibula	64
Dorsal view of wrist	32	Ankle	66
Anterior (palmar) view of left hand	34	Foot	68
Sternum	36		

Preface

This book was compiled to show diagnostic imaging technicians, medical students, trainees in diagnostic radiology and established consultants what a normal bone scan looks like, to demonstrate the amount of anatomical detail which can be seen and to a lesser extent show some areas of increased or decreased activity which are normal but may be mistaken for disease. It is in this latter area that consultant radiologists and specialists in nuclear medicine will find the book of greatest value. The reader benefits from a constant direct comparison of what is seen on the scintigraph with identical radiographs and photographs of the skeleton.

For those in training and in practice the book should prove valuable since it demonstrates normal skeletal anatomy so important in the understanding and accurate reporting of nuclear medicine scans (scintigrams).

All the images in this book were produced by the diagnostic imaging departments at Guy's Hospital, London and Pembury Hospital, Tunbridge Wells. The painstaking task of adjusting the size of the images so that they are all of comparable size was undertaken by George Kaim (Medical Photography Department, Guy's Hospital). The text and labelling was typed by my secretary, Elizabeth Mercer, with some assistance from Helen Upperton. While credit is due to many people for enabling this book to be published the aforementioned have contributed exceptional care and patience which is greatly appreciated.

I would like to thank Professor Maisey for his advice, guidance and especially for his encouragement at times when things got difficult and one was left with hundreds of images of different shapes and sizes with no end in sight. The layout of the book, i.e. the scintigram, radiograph, photograph scheme is largely due to his idea born of an understanding as to how scintigraphy might favourably be displayed and taught.

James. J. Flanagan

Anterior view of whole body

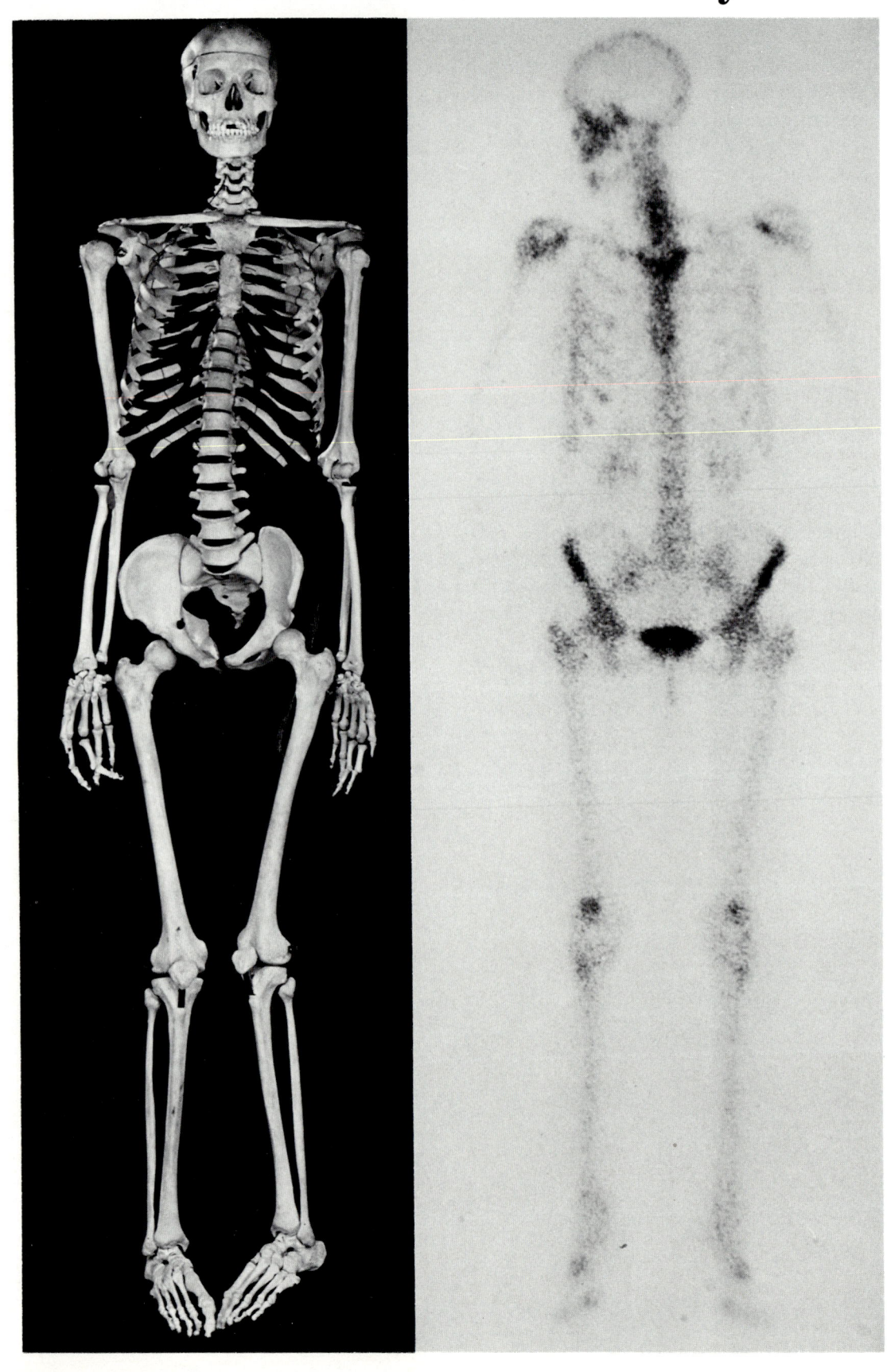

Posterior view of whole body

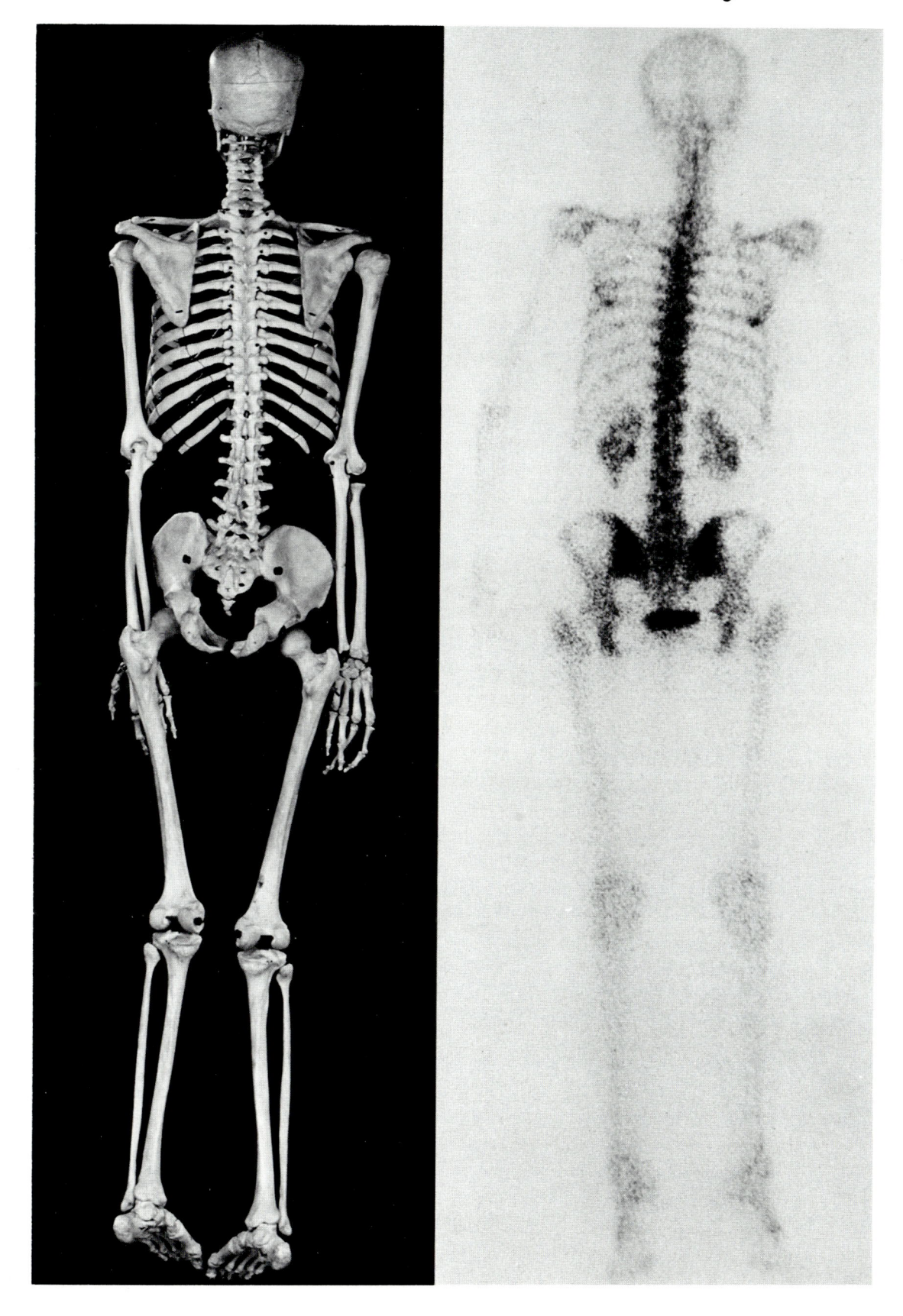

Anterior view of skull

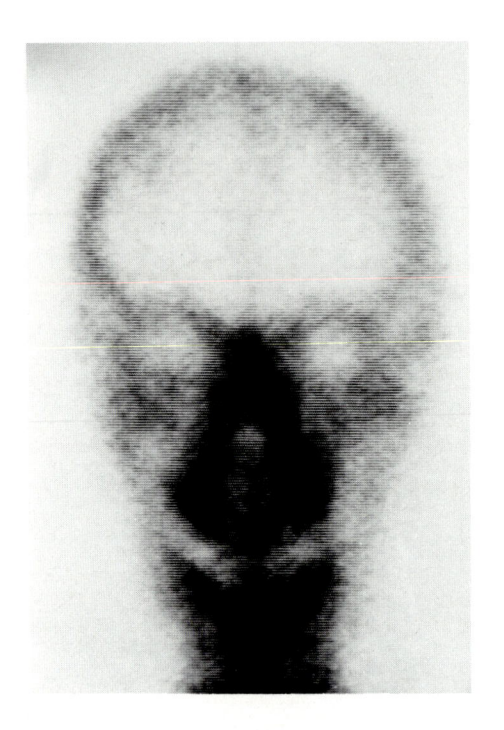

(i) The bones of the calvarium with their large diploe take up very little activity and are therefore hardly discernible when viewed 'en face'. However, in profile, due to superimposed skull tables they appear considerably more active.

(ii) The nasal and paranasal sinuses are very active.

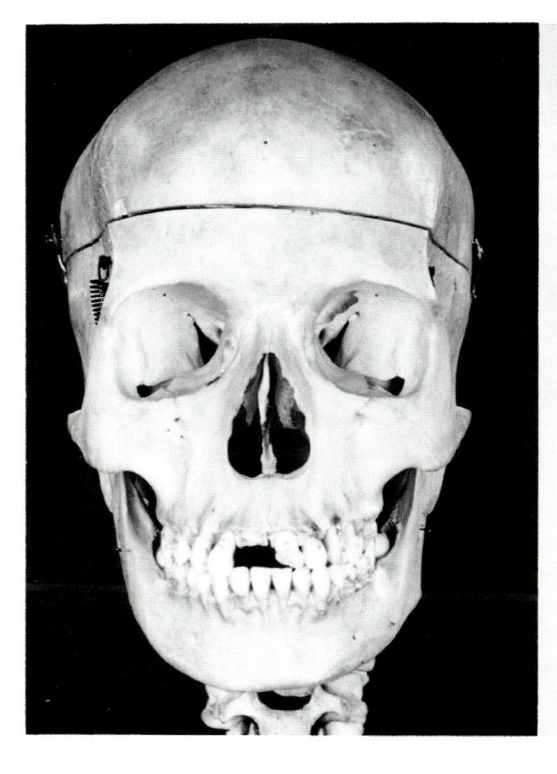

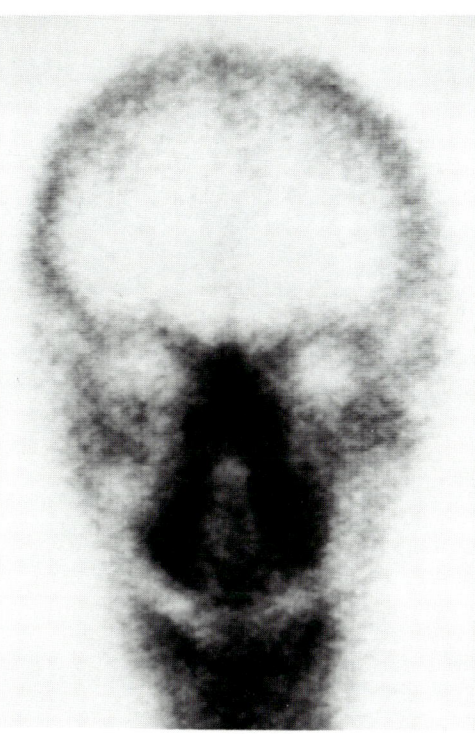

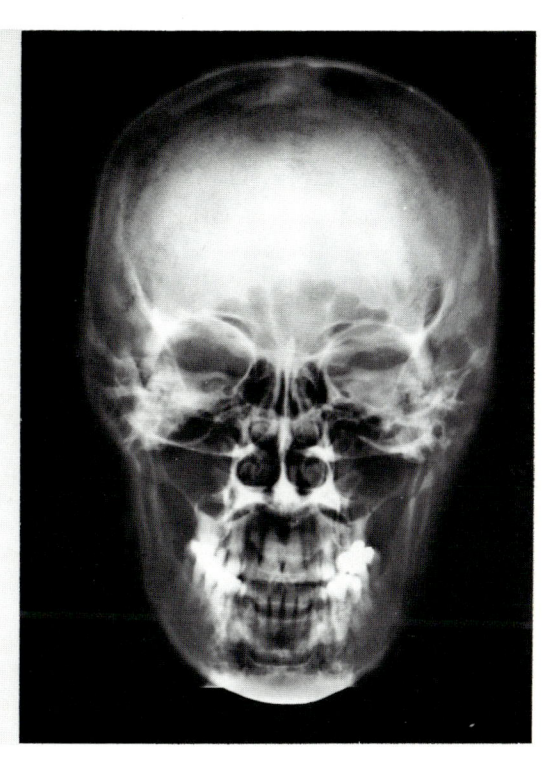

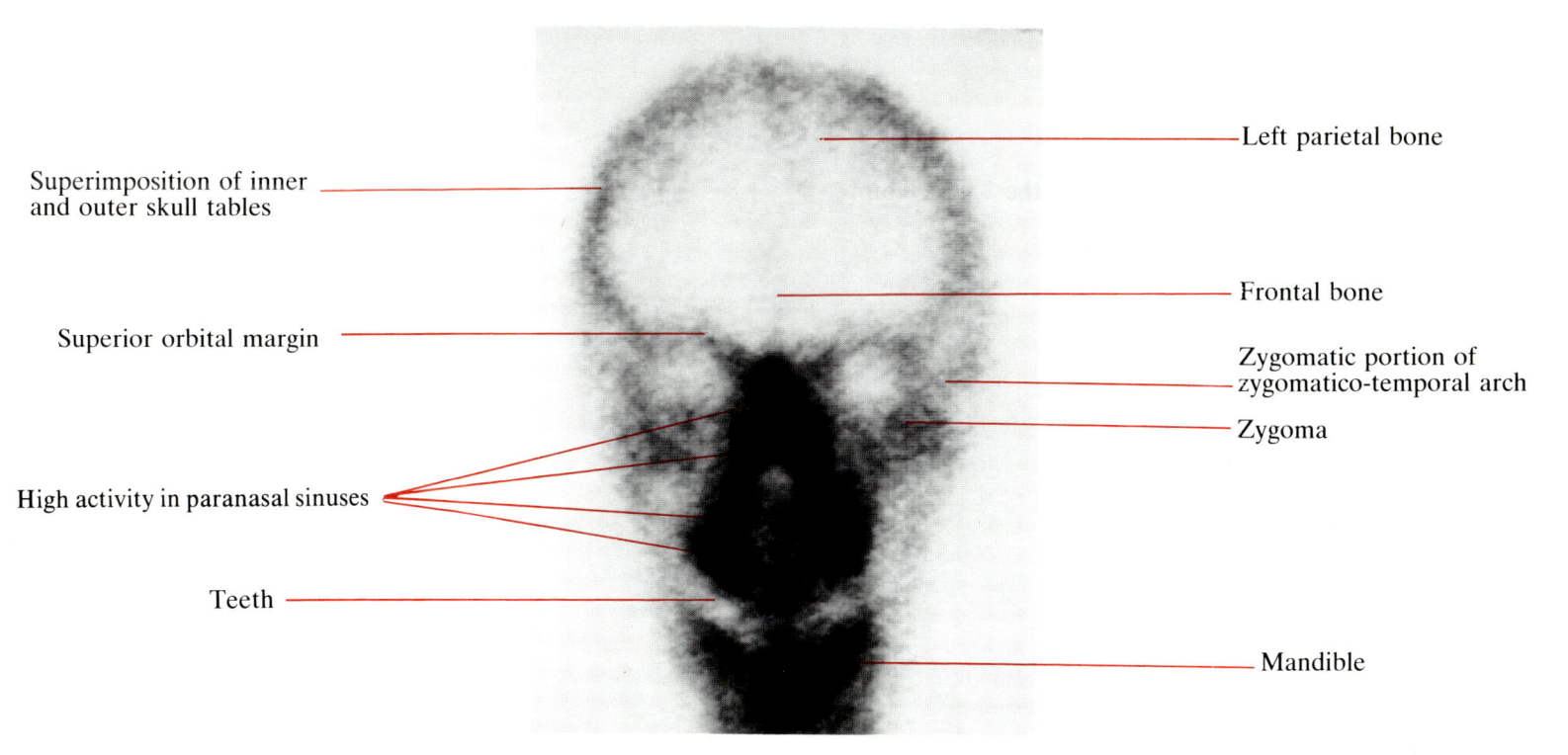

Left parietal bone

Frontal bone

Zygomatic portion of zygomatico-temporal arch

Zygoma

Mandible

Superimposition of inner and outer skull tables

Superior orbital margin

High activity in paranasal sinuses

Teeth

11

Lateral skull

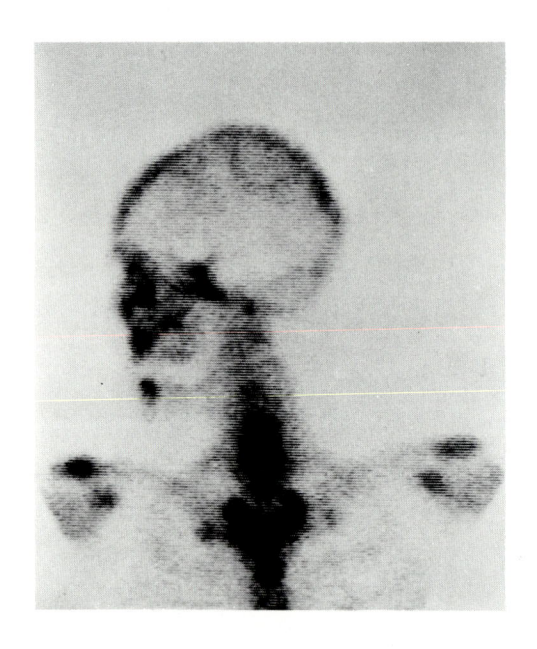

(i) Frontal sinus — the bones surrounding this structure are thin and the increased activity here may be due to mucosal rather than osseous uptake. This also applies to the nasium and maxillary antrum.

(ii) Maxilla — increased activity at this site is not seen in all patients but is so common as to be regarded as a normal finding. This also applies to the incisor area in the mandible albeit less frequent.

(iii) Base of skull and calvarium — the inner and outer skull tables are thin structures and demonstrate little activity 'en face' but due to summation of activity, appear very active when viewed tangentially.

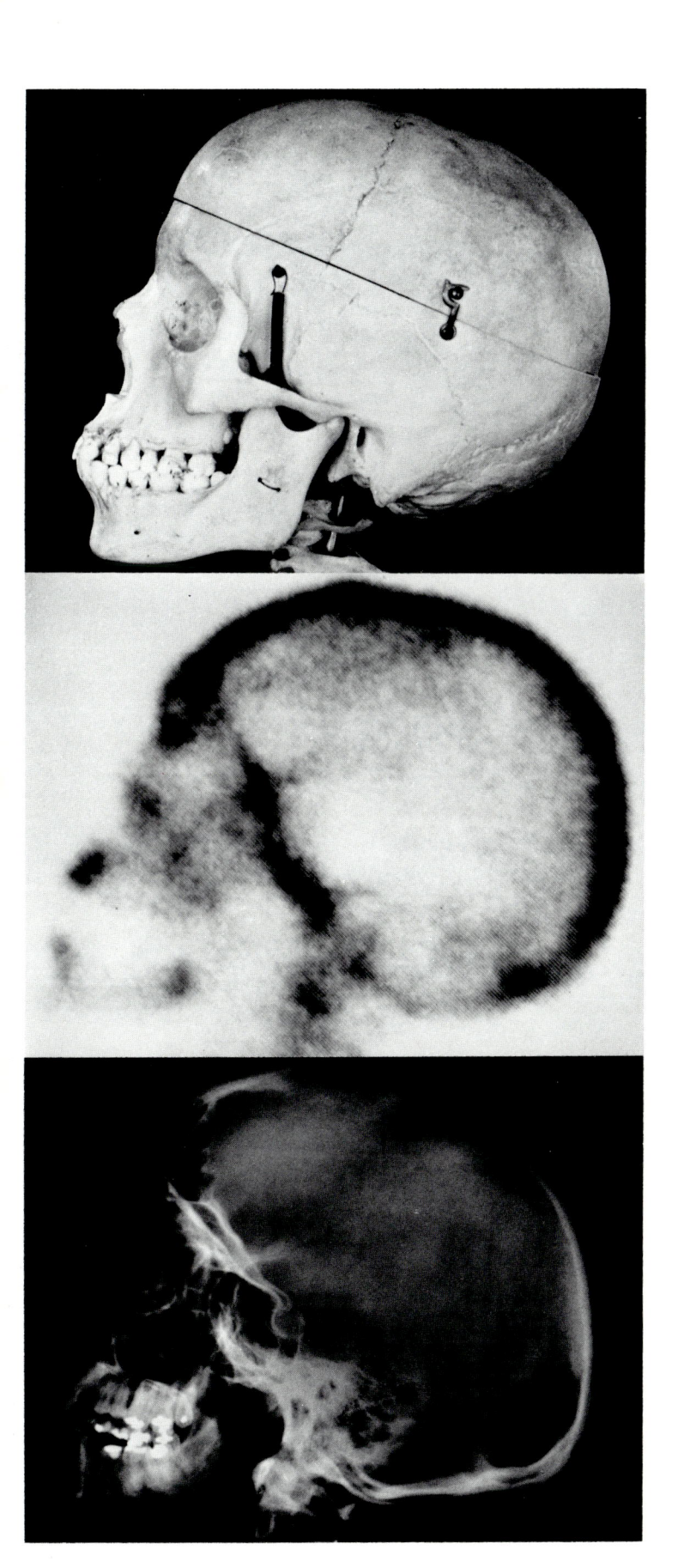

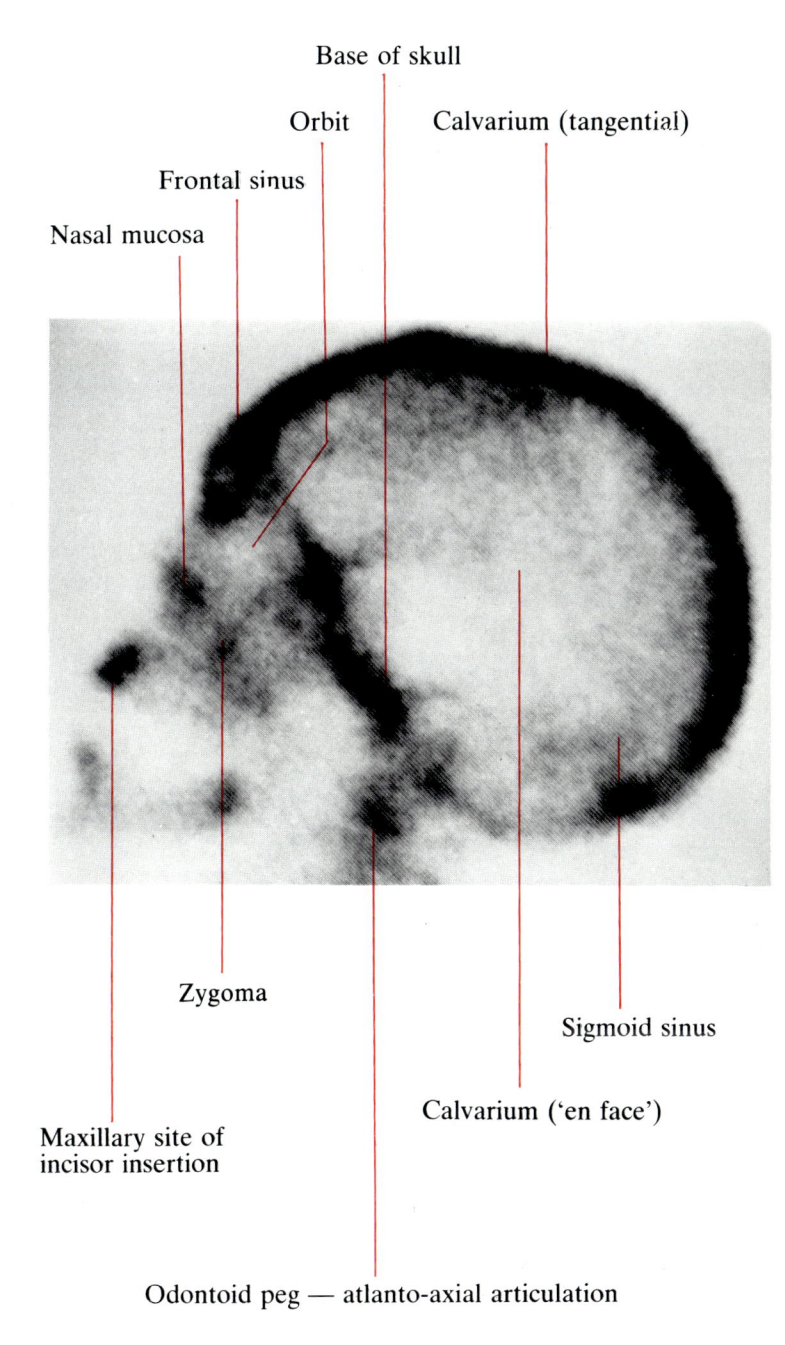

Base of skull
Orbit
Calvarium (tangential)
Frontal sinus
Nasal mucosa

Zygoma
Sigmoid sinus
Maxillary site of incisor insertion
Calvarium ('en face')
Odontoid peg — atlanto-axial articulation

Turned oblique view of cervical spine

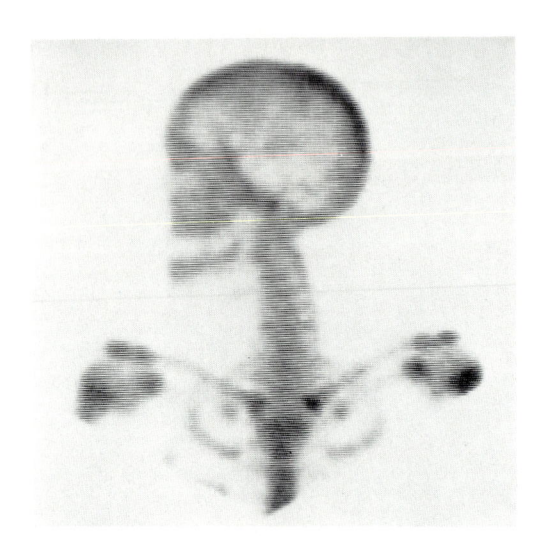

(i) It is not possible in most departments to get the large gamma camera sufficiently close to the cervical spine for a lateral view. Therefore, as illustrated here, a compromise is achieved i.e. the turned lateral view. There is no corresponding radiographic view of the cervical spine and the nearest comparable view would be a lateral or oblique radiograph. In this case the former has been chosen.

(ii) It follows from (i) that the demonstrated anatomy will vary with the obliquity of the spine e.g. a transverse process may be seen in the lowermost or least turned portion, whereas this is not apparent in the upper spine which is the most lateral portion. Between these points maximum obliquity allows an intervertebral foramen to be clearly seen.

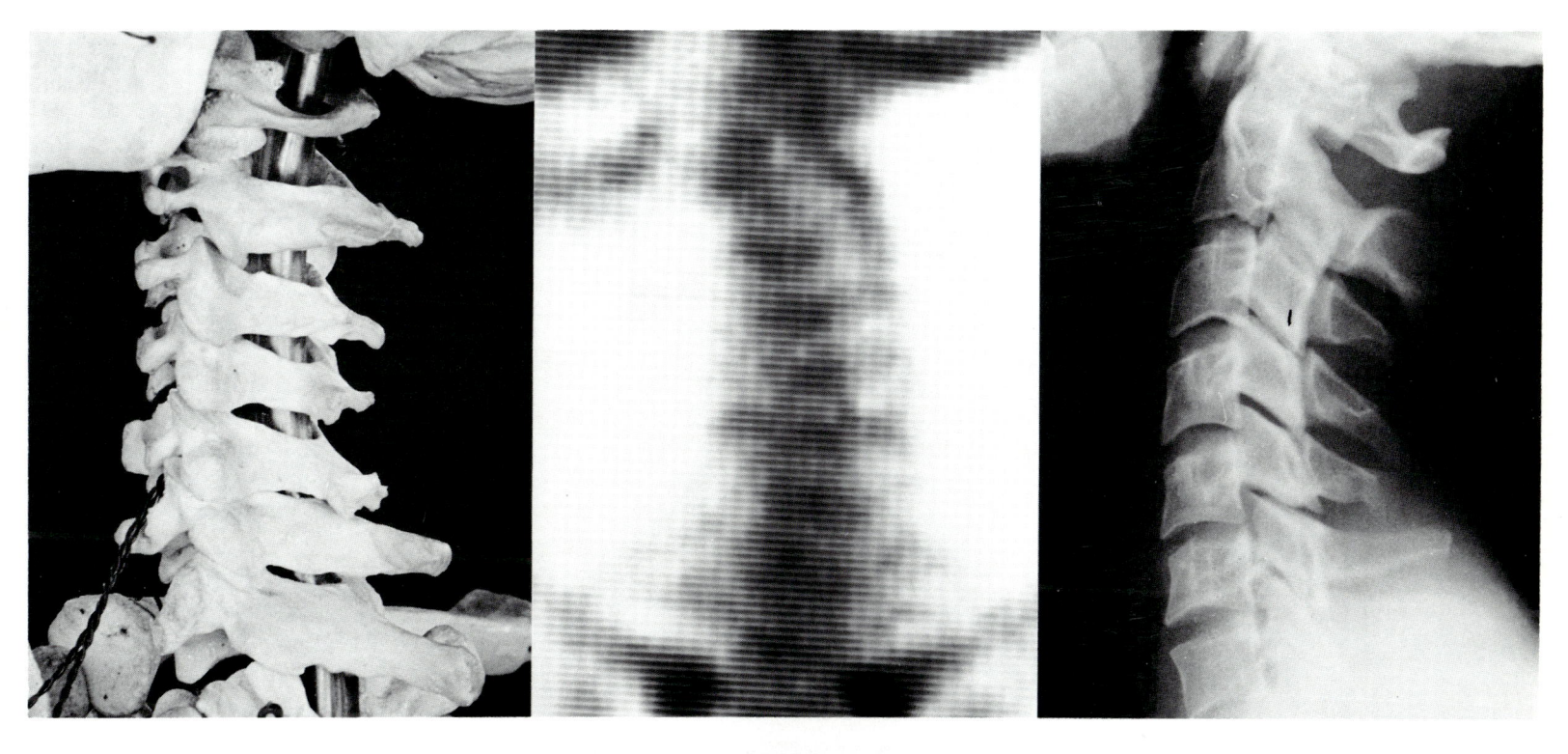

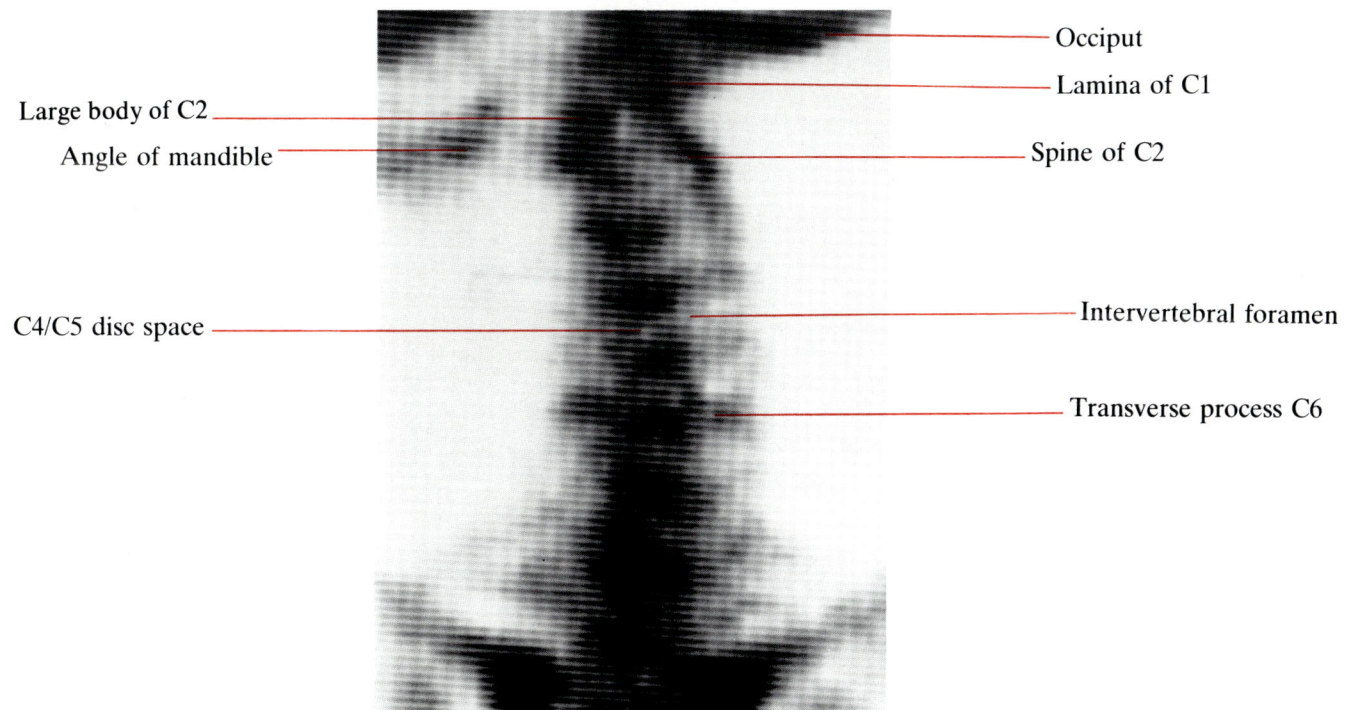

Occiput

Lamina of C1

Large body of C2

Angle of mandible

Spine of C2

C4/C5 disc space

Intervertebral foramen

Transverse process C6

Posterior view of cervical spine

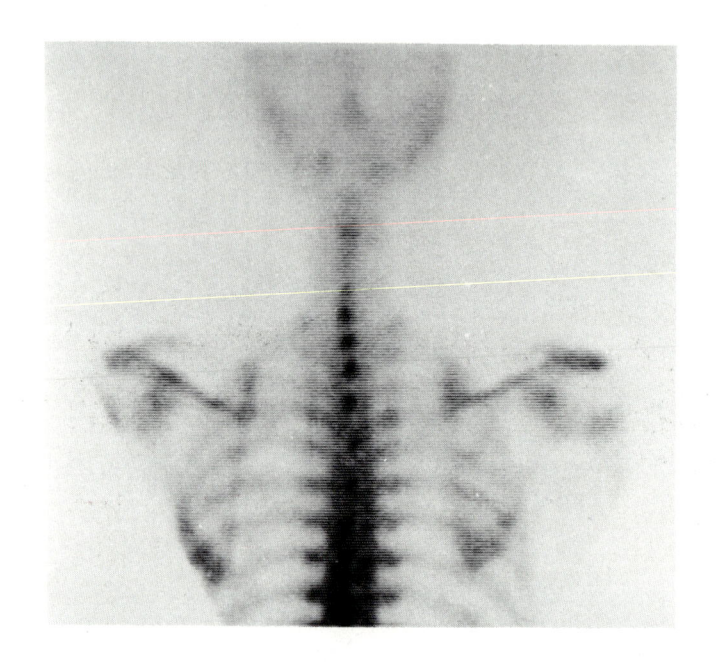

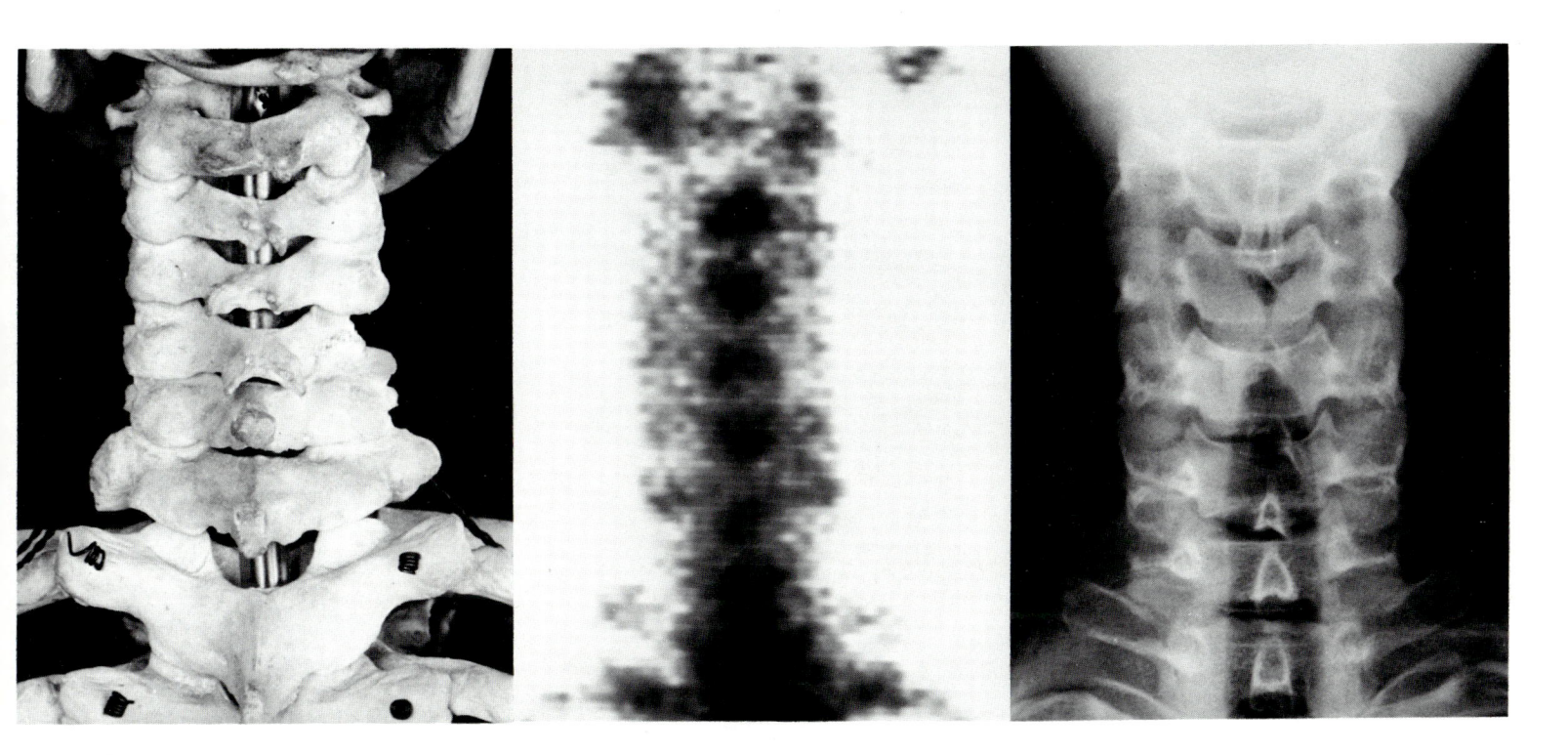

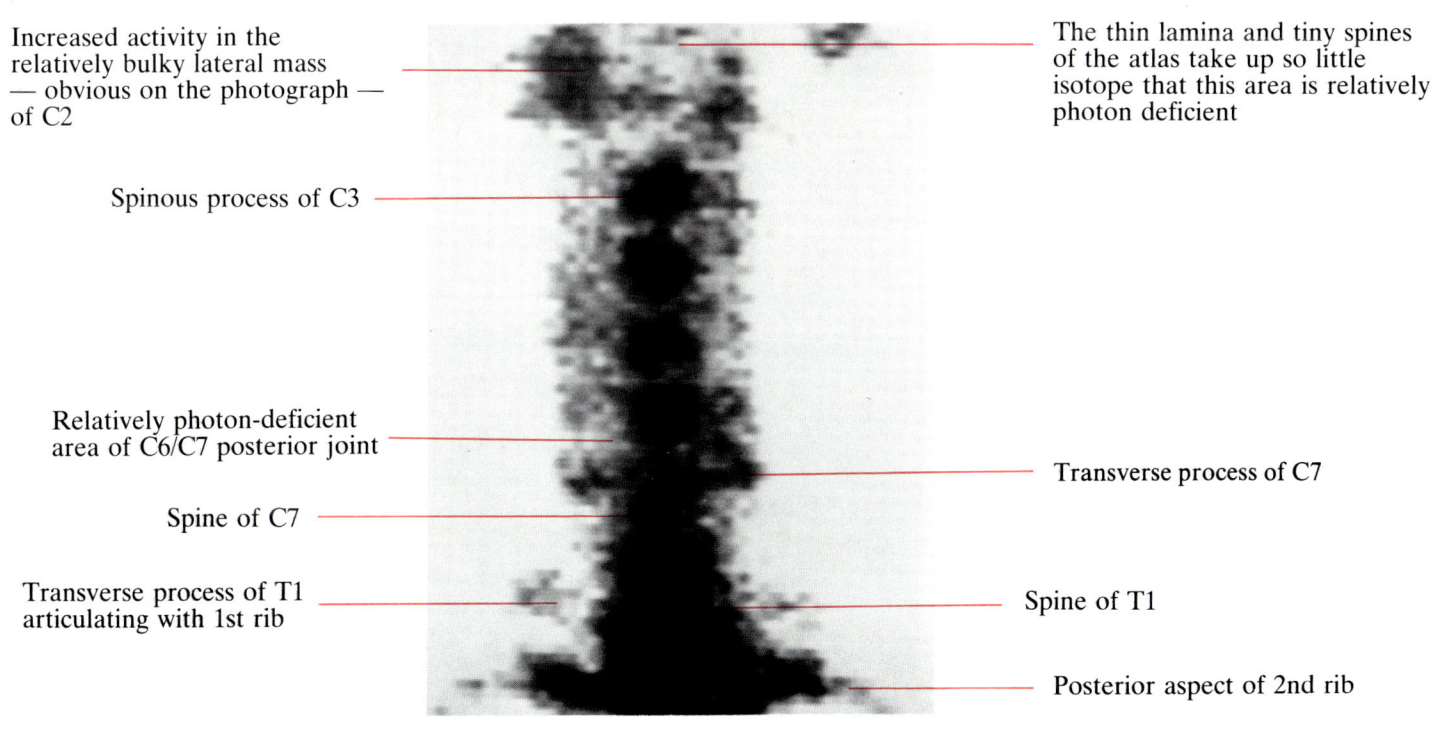

Increased activity in the relatively bulky lateral mass — obvious on the photograph — of C2

Spinous process of C3

Relatively photon-deficient area of C6/C7 posterior joint

Spine of C7

Transverse process of T1 articulating with 1st rib

The thin lamina and tiny spines of the atlas take up so little isotope that this area is relatively photon deficient

Transverse process of C7

Spine of T1

Posterior aspect of 2nd rib

Anterior view of clavicle

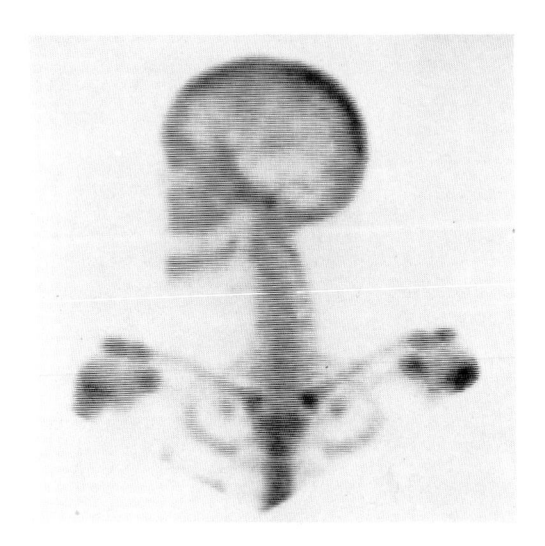

(i) The rather S shaped anatomy of this bone can be better appreciated from the scintigram than any of the other images. As its medial portion bows anteriorly it appears as an area of relatively increased activity only to almost disappear as it courses posteriorly in its lateral middle third, here it becomes more active as the final portion of the S draws anteriorly to make the acromioclavicular joint.

Acromioclavicular joint

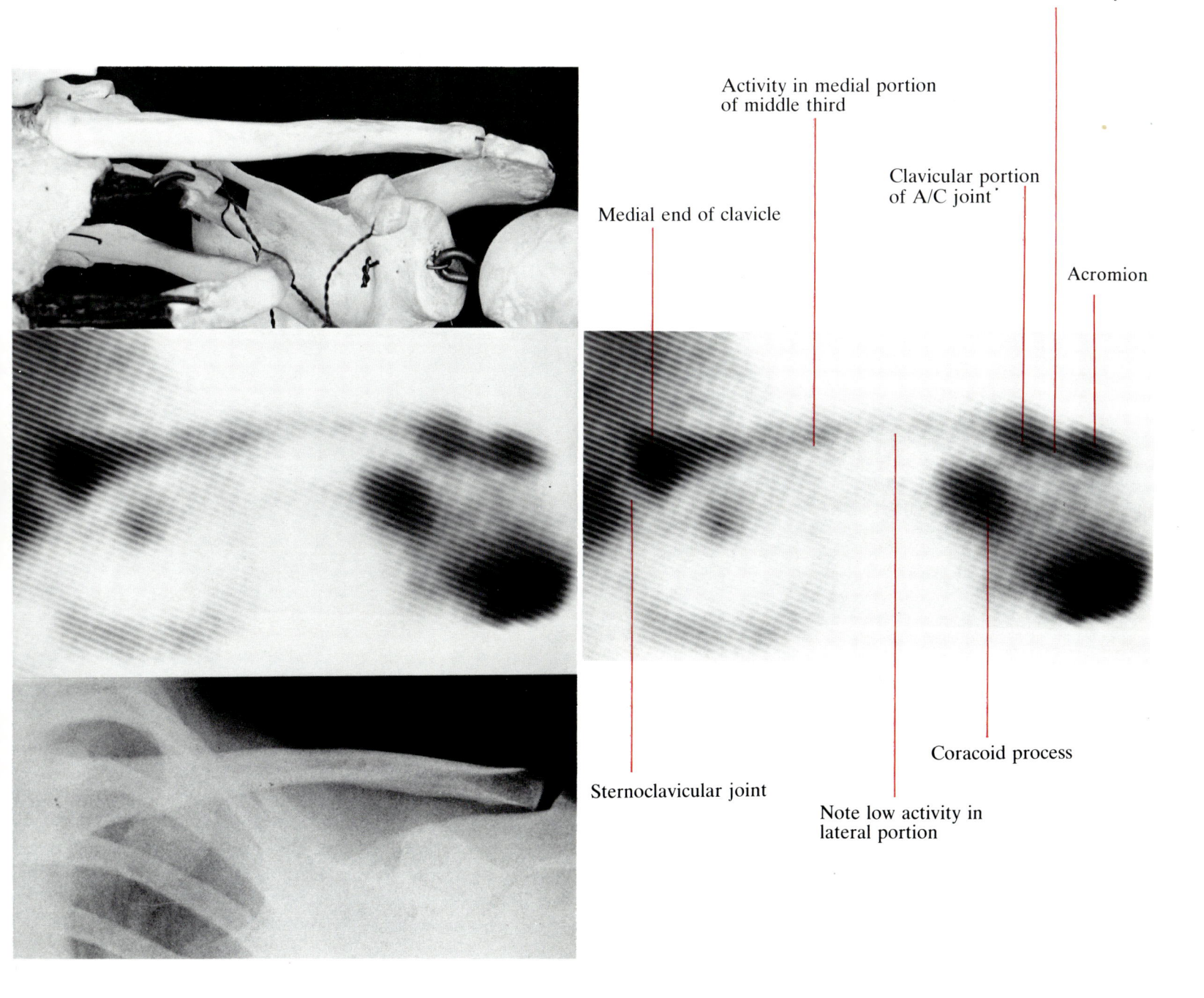

Activity in medial portion of middle third

Clavicular portion of A/C joint

Medial end of clavicle

Acromion

Sternoclavicular joint

Note low activity in lateral portion

Coracoid process

Anterior view of left shoulder

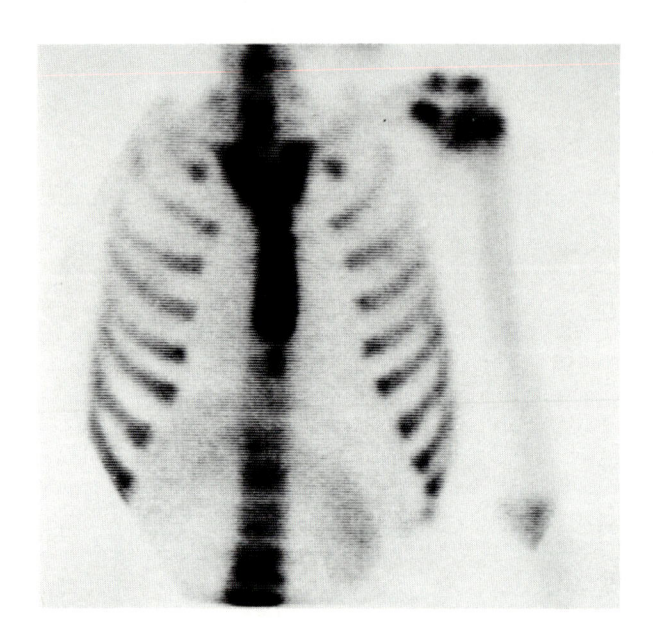

(i) Increased activity in the relatively small structure of the coracoid process belies its anterior position. Identification of this (and other) structures may thus indicate the position in which the patient was scanned.

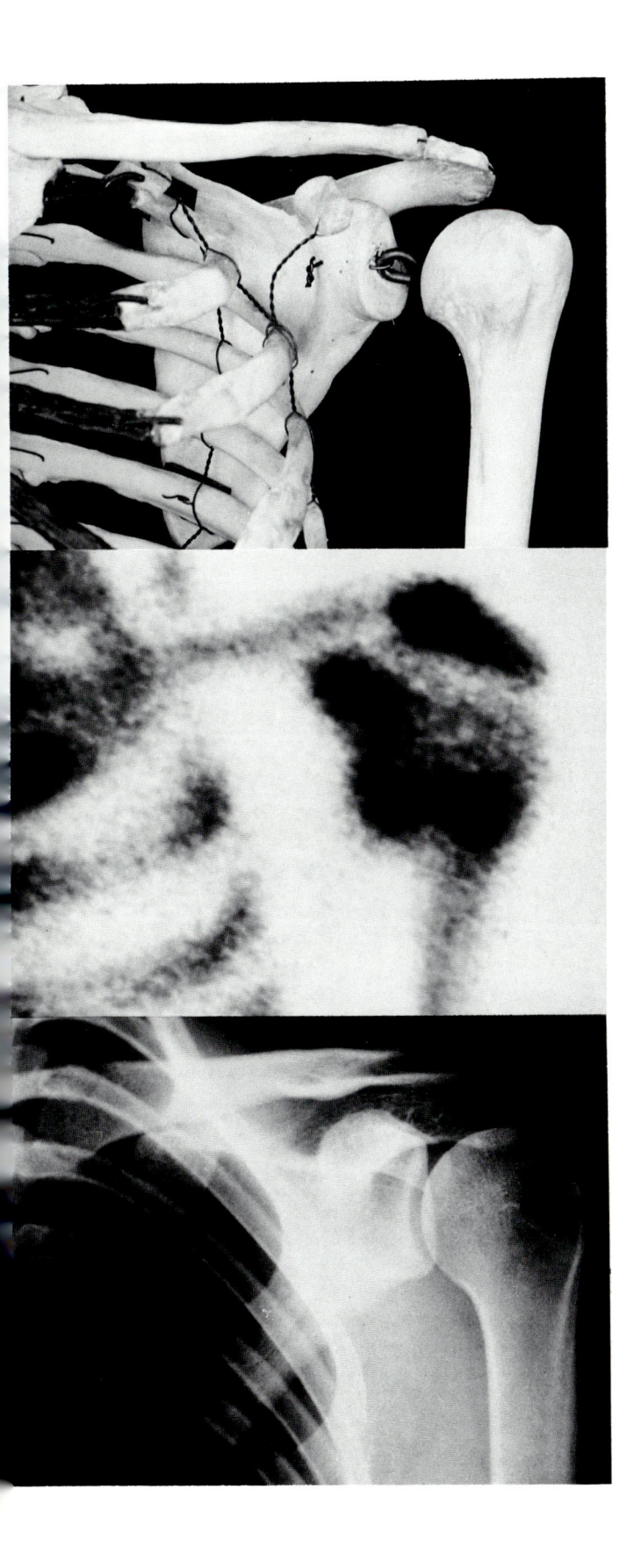

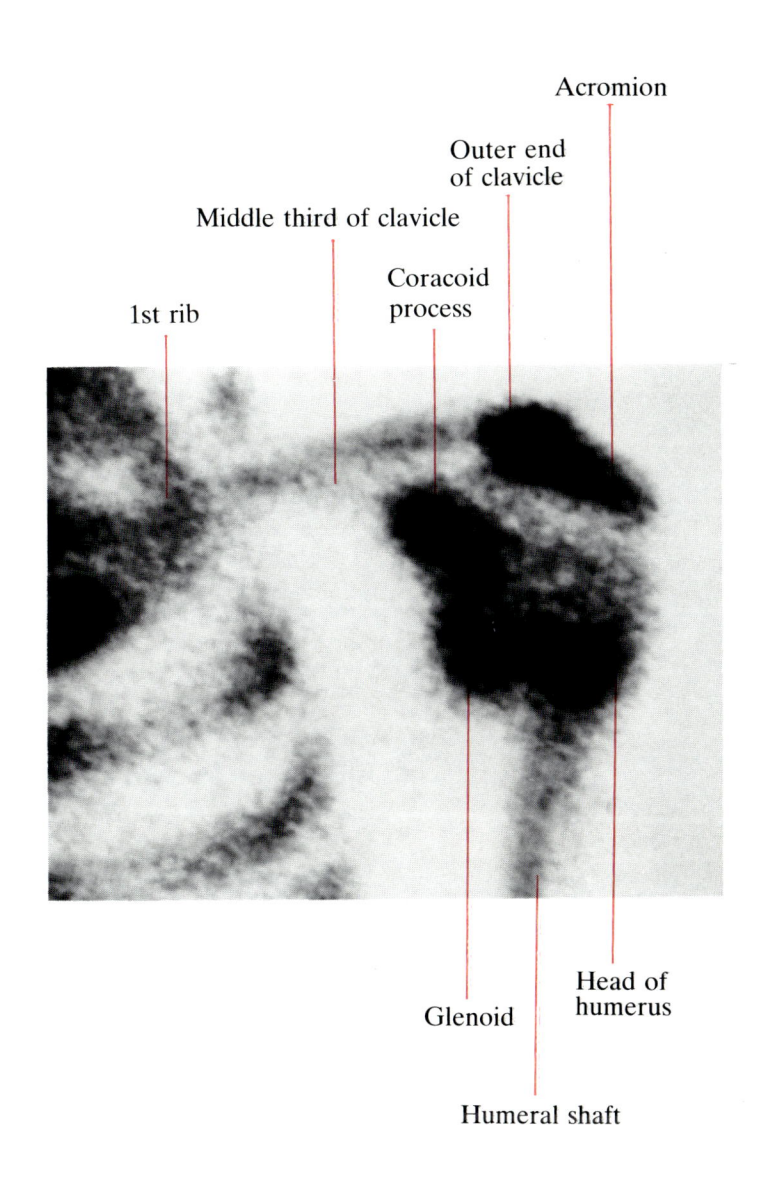

Acromion

Outer end
of clavicle

Middle third of clavicle

Coracoid
process

1st rib

Glenoid

Head of
humerus

Humeral shaft

21

Posterior view of scapula

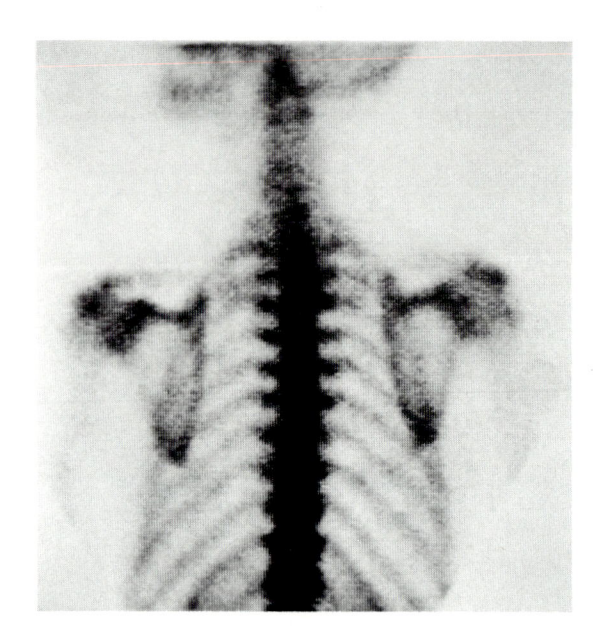

(i) The thinner parts of the bone, e.g. the superior angle and lateral border take up so little tracer that they cannot be visualised.

(ii) The lateral aspect of the spine has increased activity due to superimposition of the coracoid process. This may be clearly understood from the photograph where the coracoid process can be seen protruding over this structure.

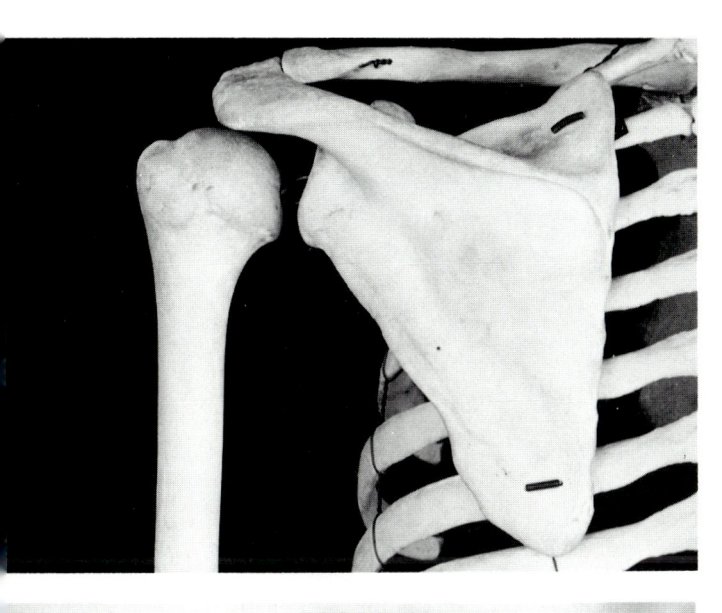

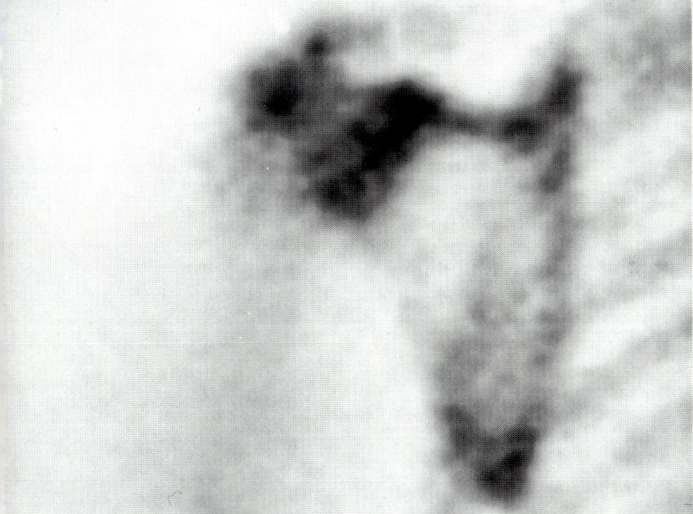

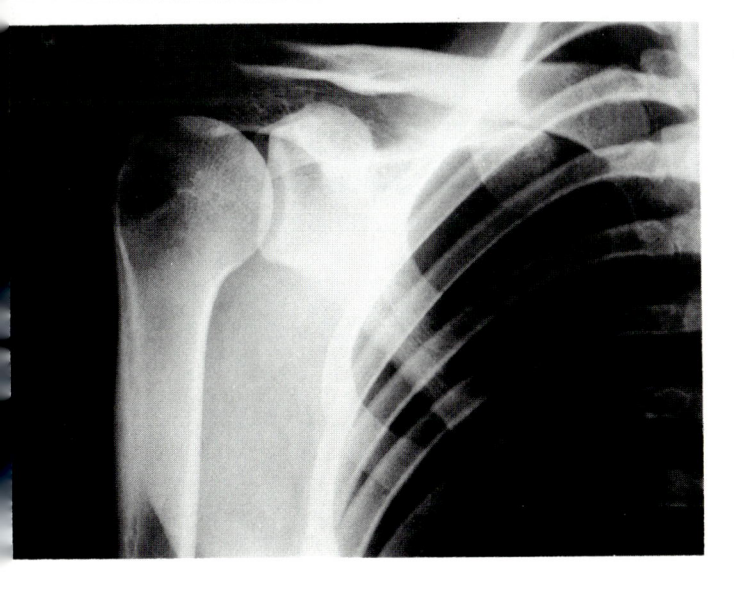

Spine with superimposed coracoid

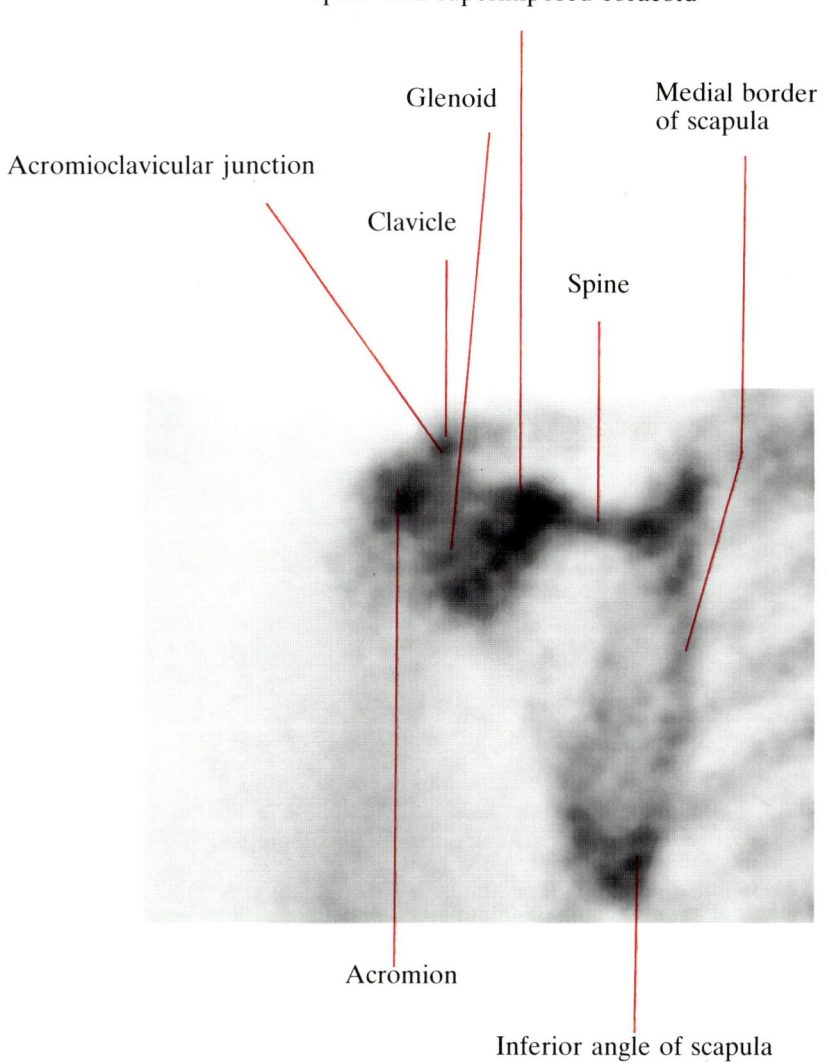

Glenoid

Medial border of scapula

Acromioclavicular junction

Clavicle

Spine

Acromion

Inferior angle of scapula

23

Anterior view of left humerus

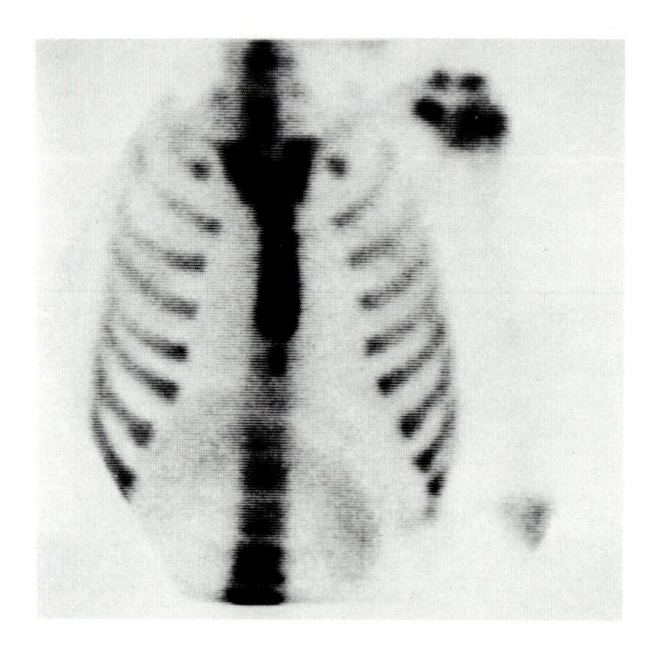

(i) Some radioactive tracer has leaked through the wall of a vein in the antecubital fossa and is seen as an area of increased activity in the soft tissues. This is a common finding if it is looked for.

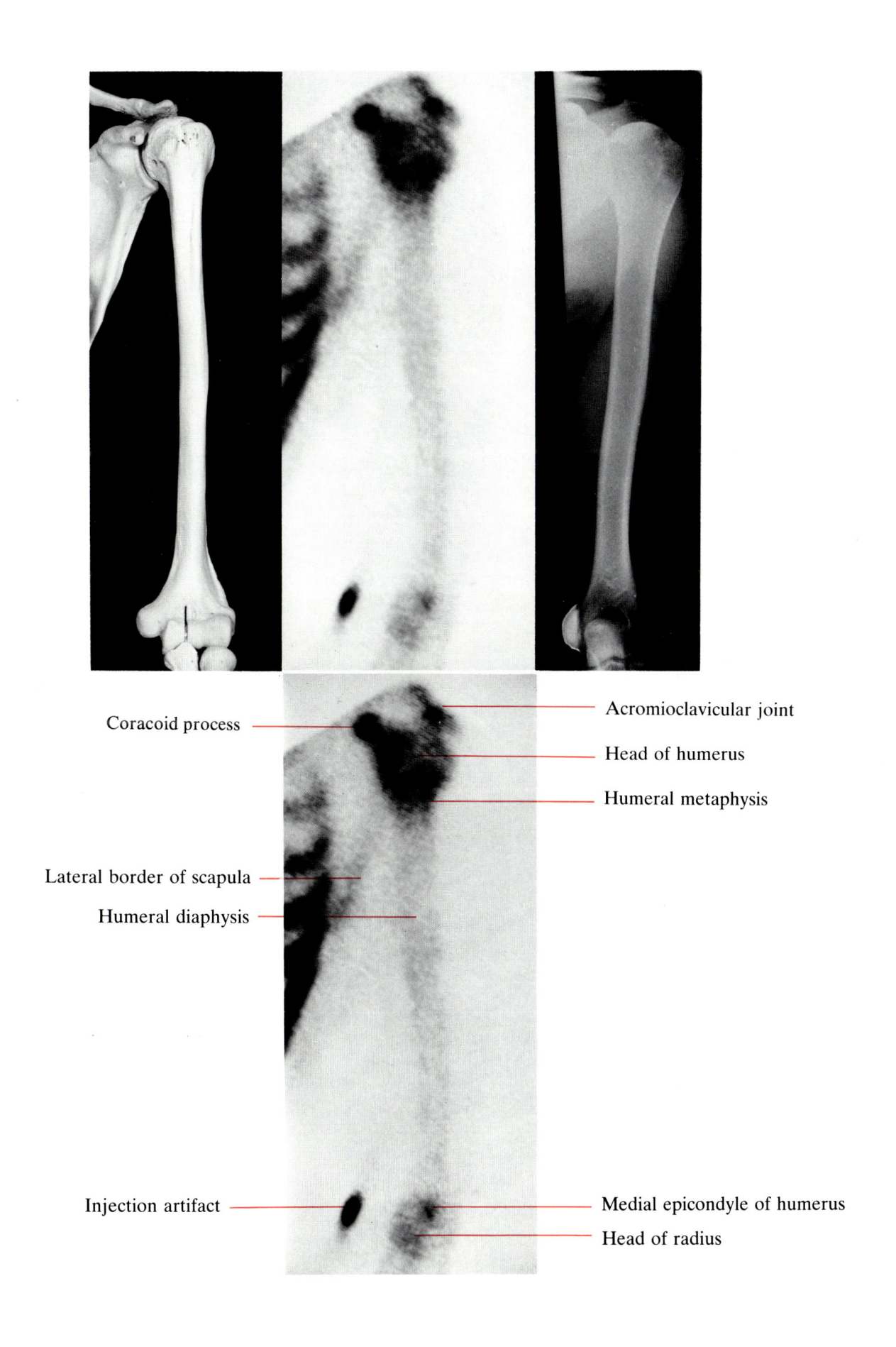

Coracoid process — Acromioclavicular joint
Head of humerus
Humeral metaphysis
Lateral border of scapula
Humeral diaphysis
Injection artifact — Medial epicondyle of humerus
Head of radius

25

Anterior view of elbow joint

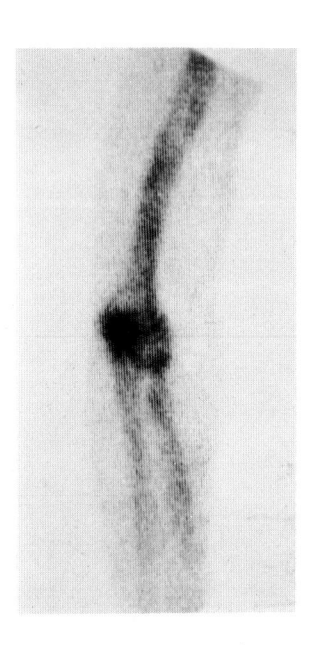

(i) Trochlea, coronoid process — the angled C shape configuration of this joint does not allow visualisation of the joint 'space'.

(ii) Ulnar diaphysis — the morphology of thin bones such as this results in low activity and consequent poor visualisation.

Humeral diaphysis

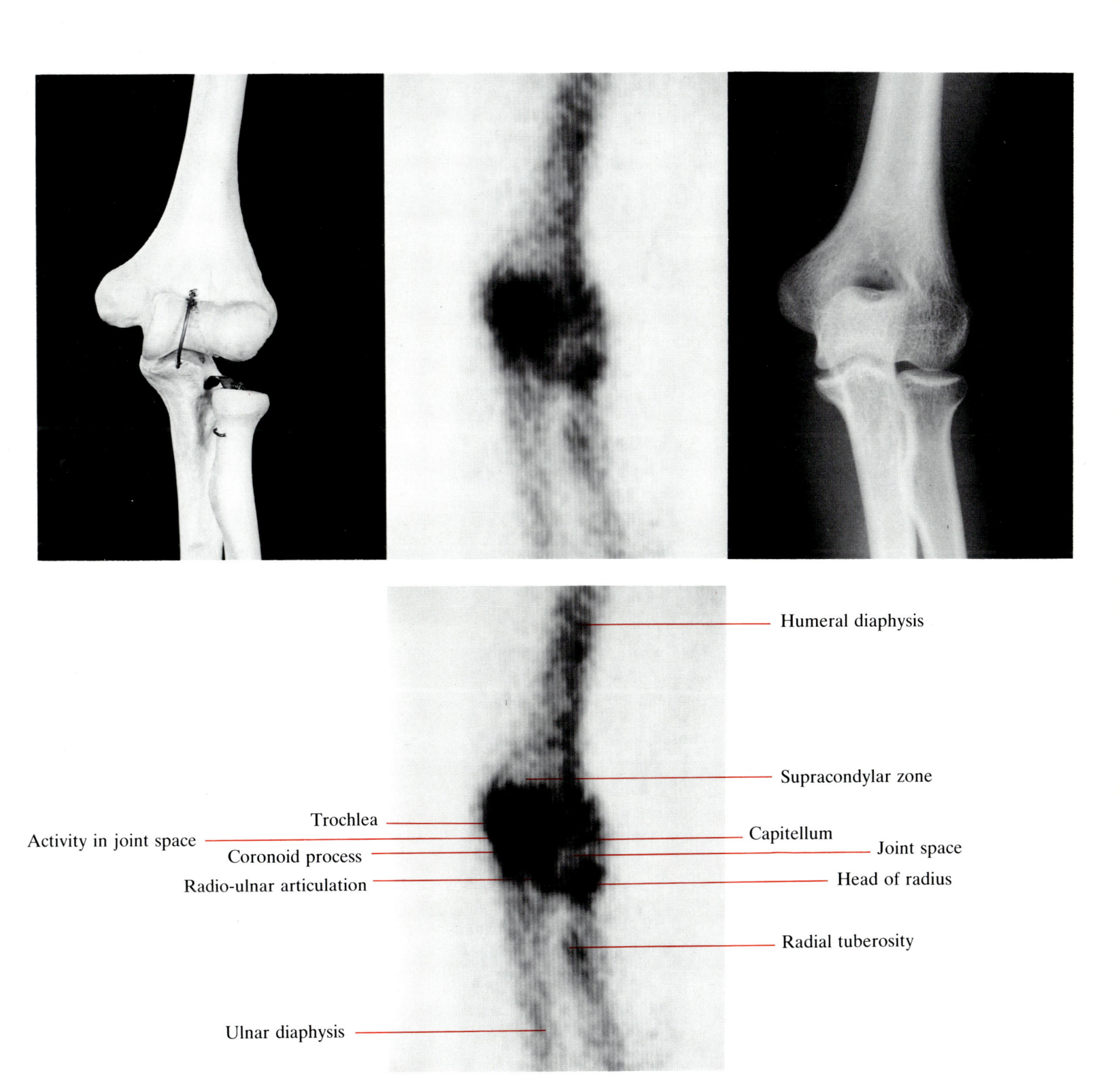

Supracondylar zone

Activity in joint space
Trochlea
Coronoid process
Radio-ulnar articulation

Capitellum
Joint space
Head of radius

Radial tuberosity

Ulnar diaphysis

27

Lateral view of elbow

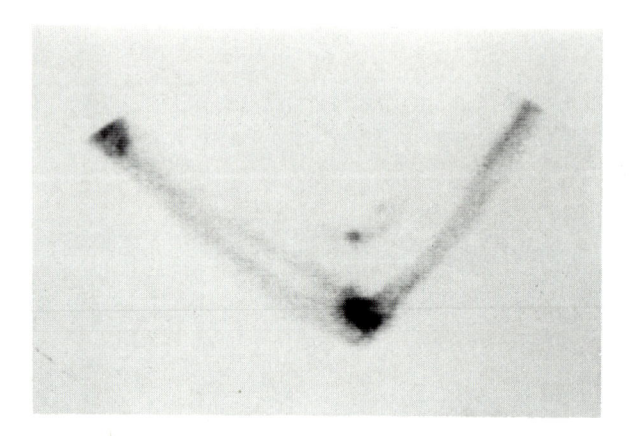

(i) The joint space is not visualised on any of the images here. This is due to the anatomical configuration of the joint whereby slight obliquity of the capitellum and trochlea do not allow photons x-rays or a light beam to pass tangential to those structures.

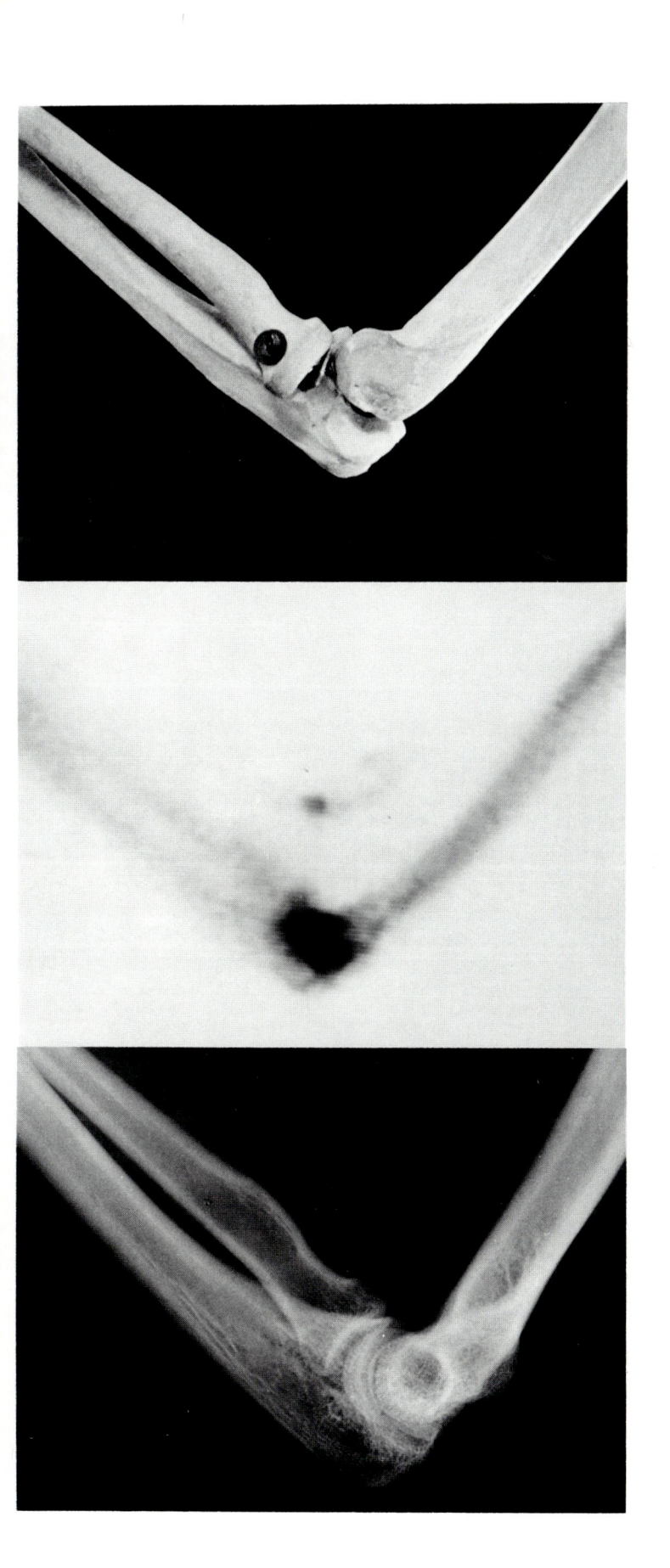

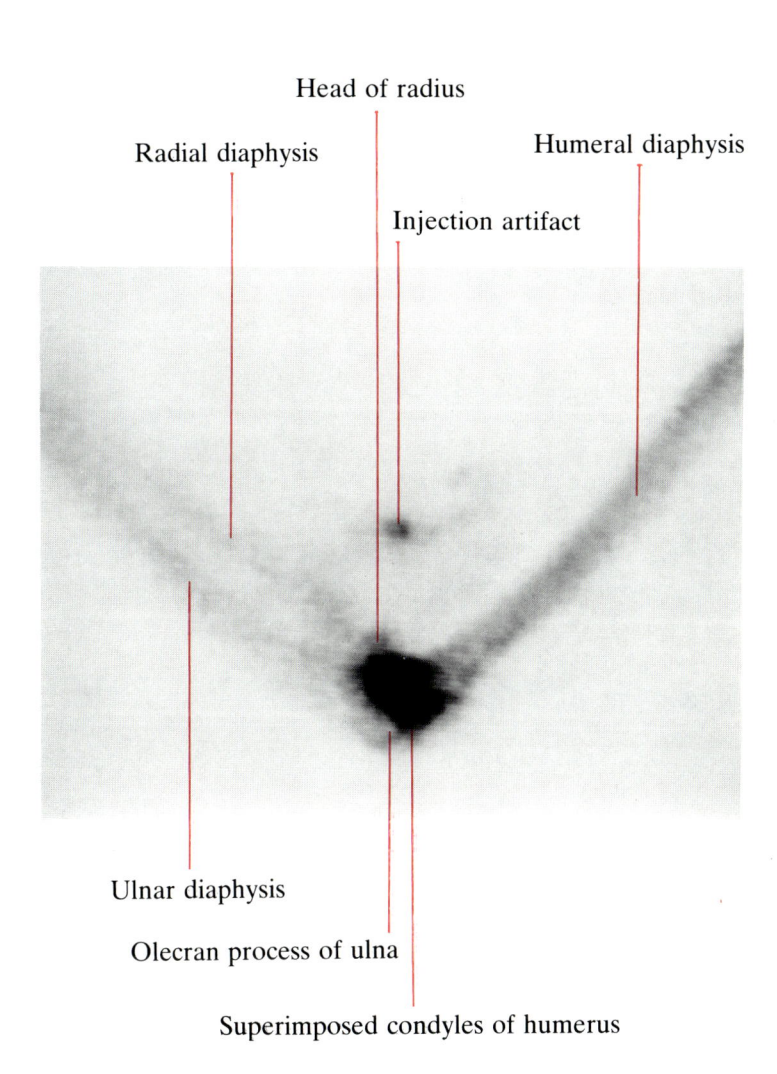

Head of radius

Radial diaphysis

Humeral diaphysis

Injection artifact

Ulnar diaphysis

Olecran process of ulna

Superimposed condyles of humerus

Anterior view of forearm

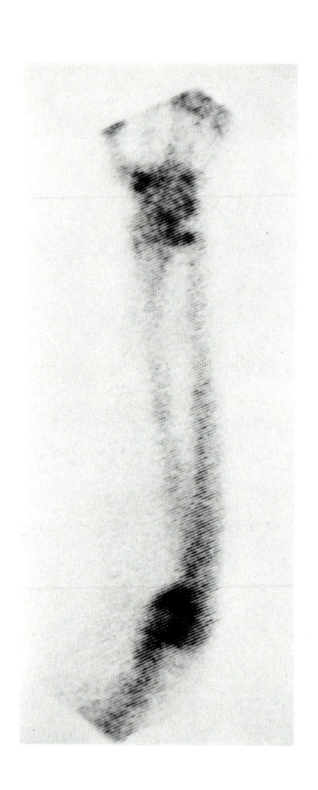

Radial metaphysis —————— Inferior radio-ulnar joint

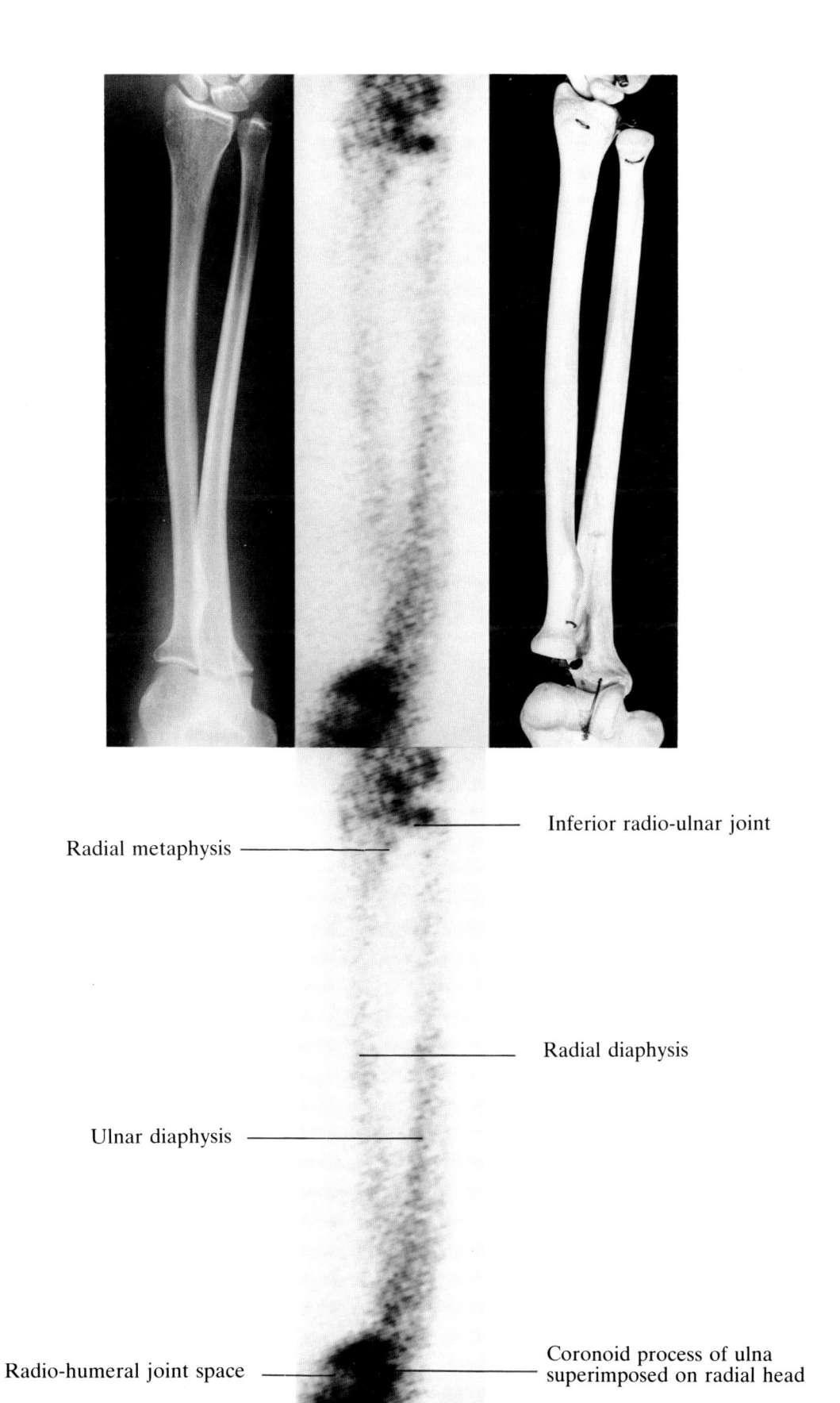

—————— Radial diaphysis

Ulnar diaphysis ——————

Radio-humeral joint space —————— Coronoid process of ulna superimposed on radial head

Dorsal view of wrist

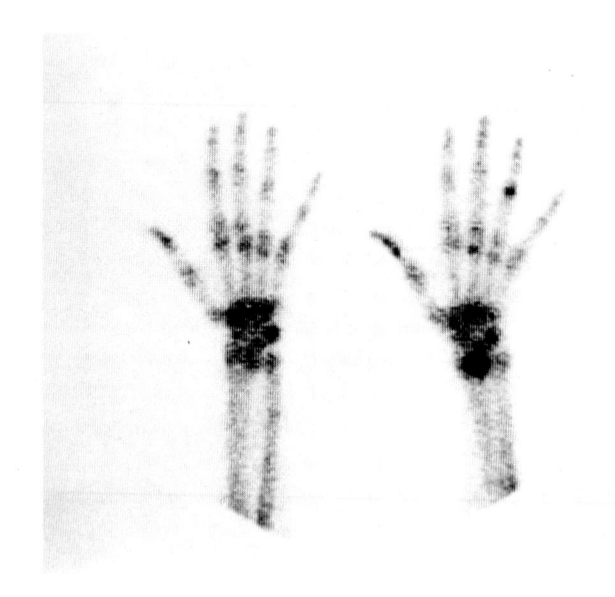

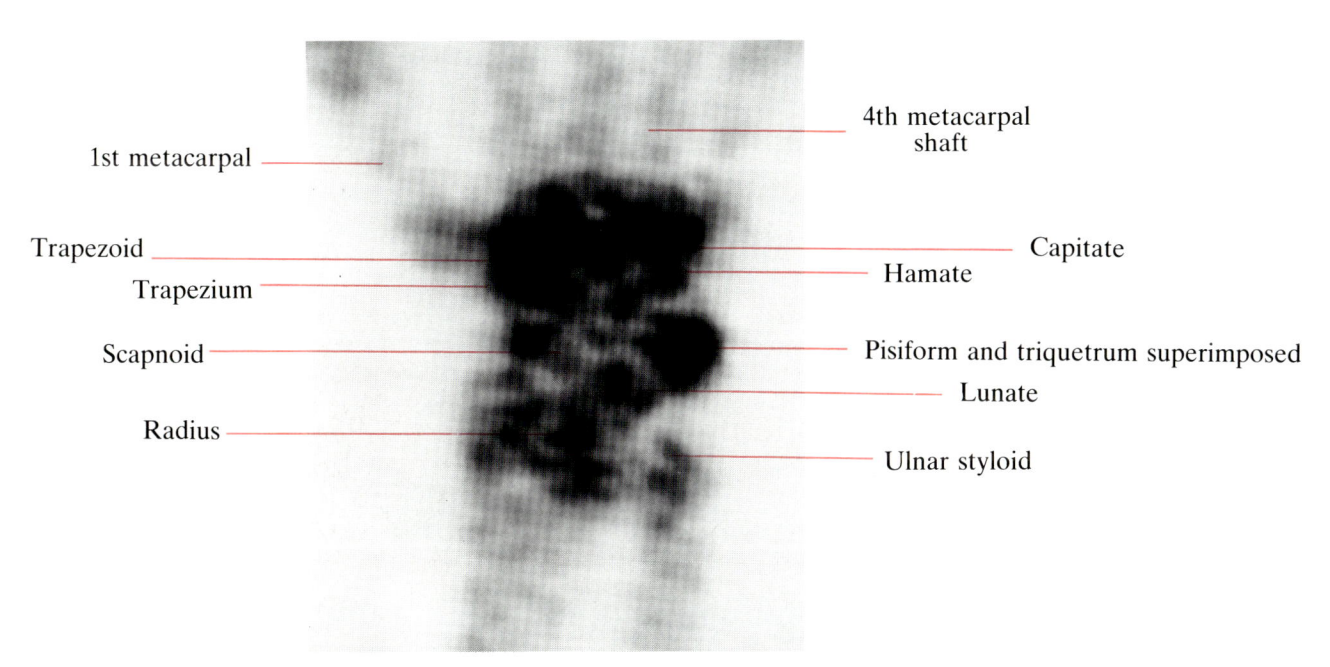

1st metacarpal —— —— 4th metacarpal shaft

Trapezoid —— —— Capitate
Trapezium —— —— Hamate

Scapnoid —— —— Pisiform and triquetrum superimposed
—— Lunate
Radius ——
—— Ulnar styloid

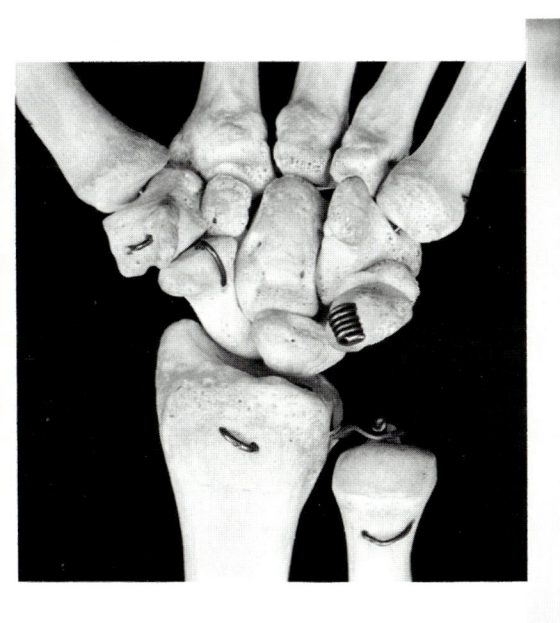

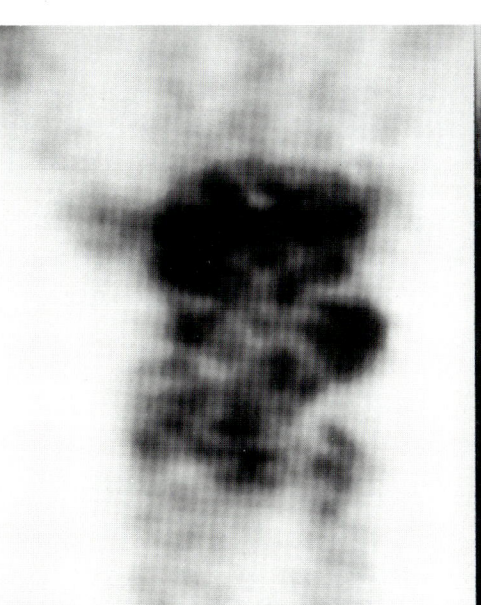

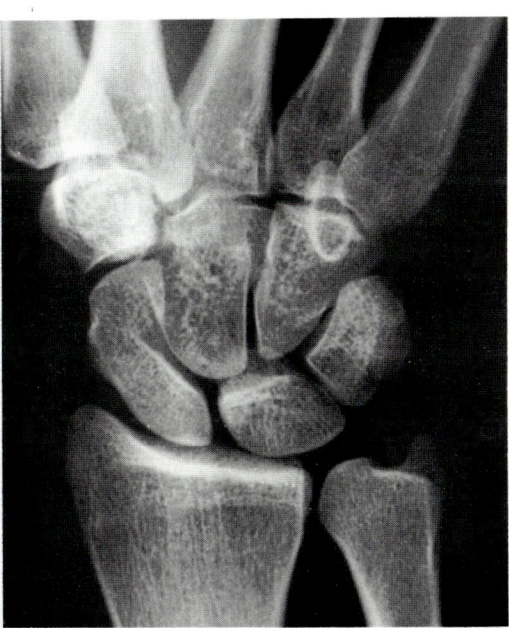

33

Anterior (Palmar) view of left hand

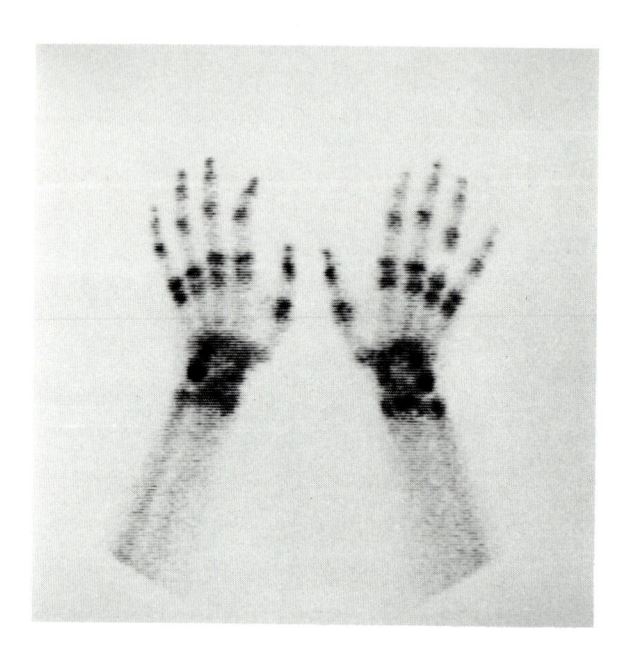

(i) This patient had not yet completely fused his epiphysis hence the increased activity at the ends of the long bones.

(ii) Because the carpal bones are in such close proximity, activity from one bone overlaps with another making precise delineation of these structures impossible at the present time.

Distal phalynx of ring finger

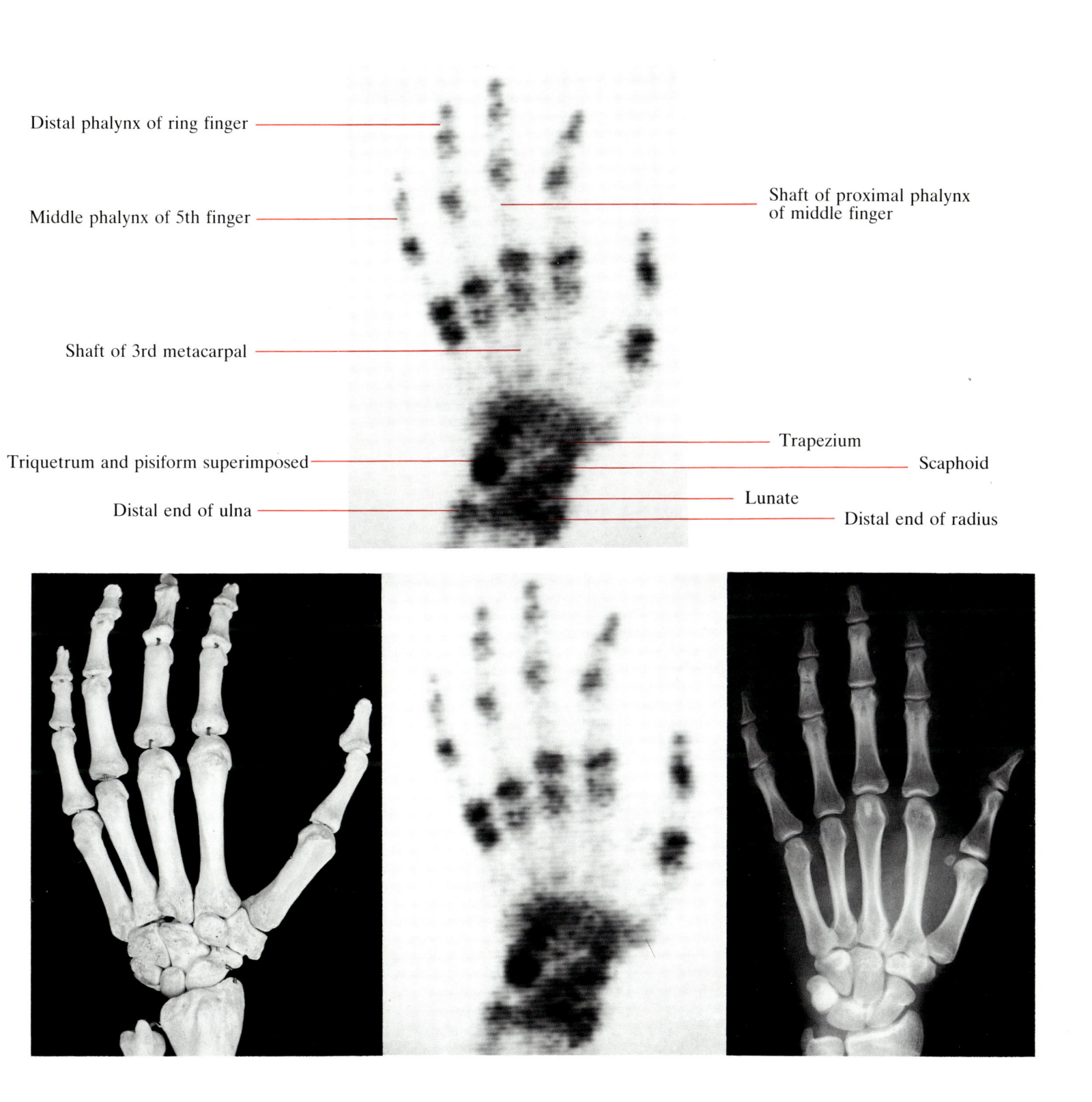

Middle phalynx of 5th finger

Shaft of proximal phalynx of middle finger

Shaft of 3rd metacarpal

Triquetrum and pisiform superimposed

Trapezium

Scaphoid

Distal end of ulna

Lunate

Distal end of radius

35

Sternum

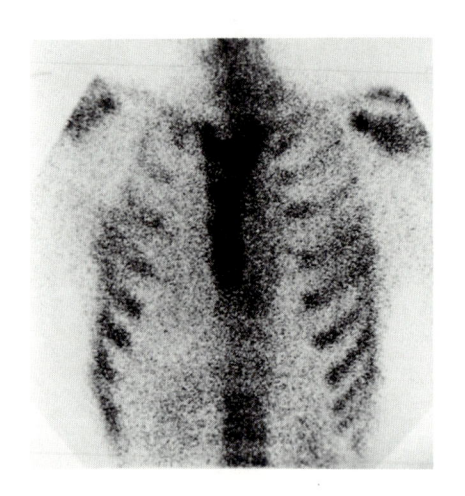

Manubrium sterni

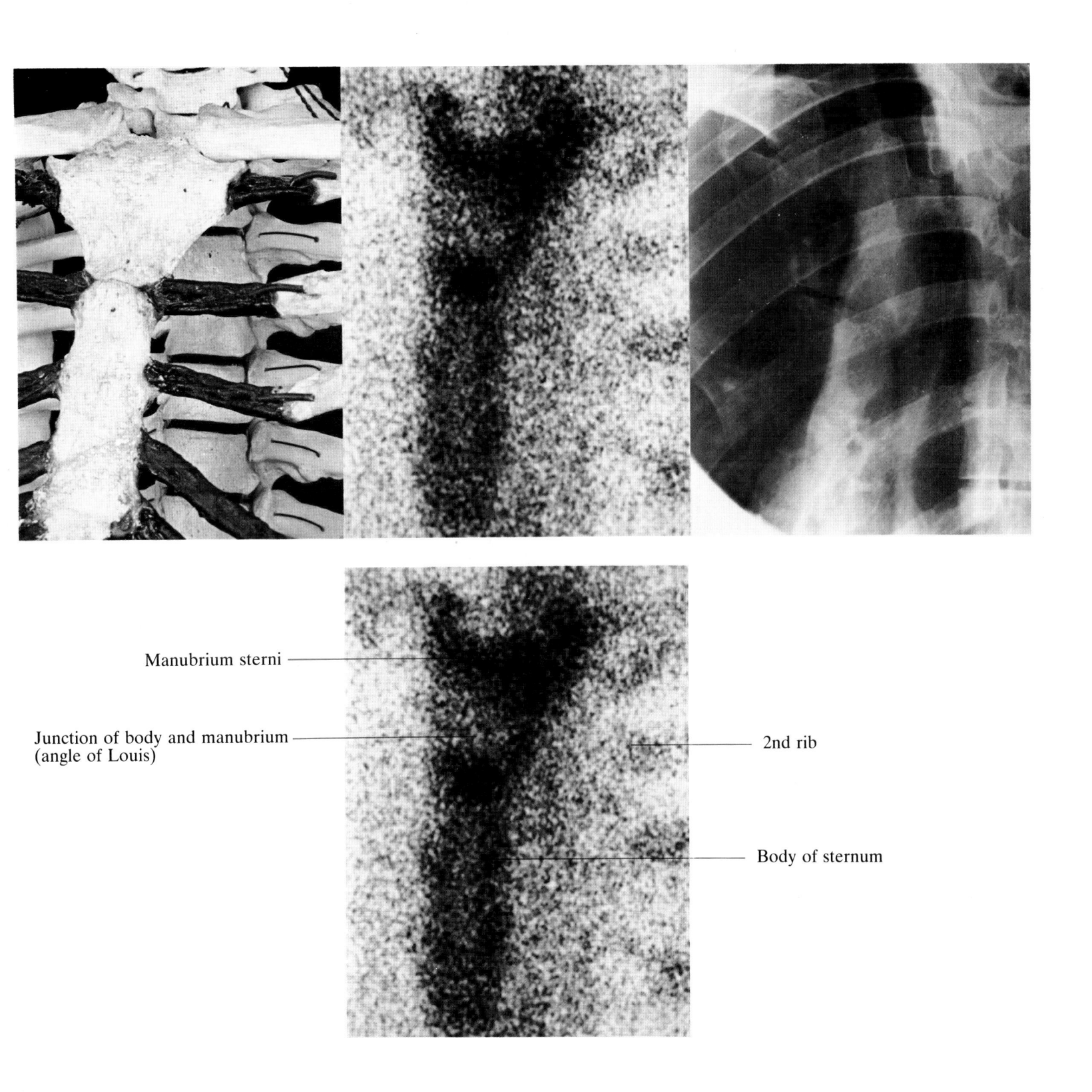

Junction of body and manubrium (angle of Louis)

2nd rib

Body of sternum

Anterior view of thoracic cage

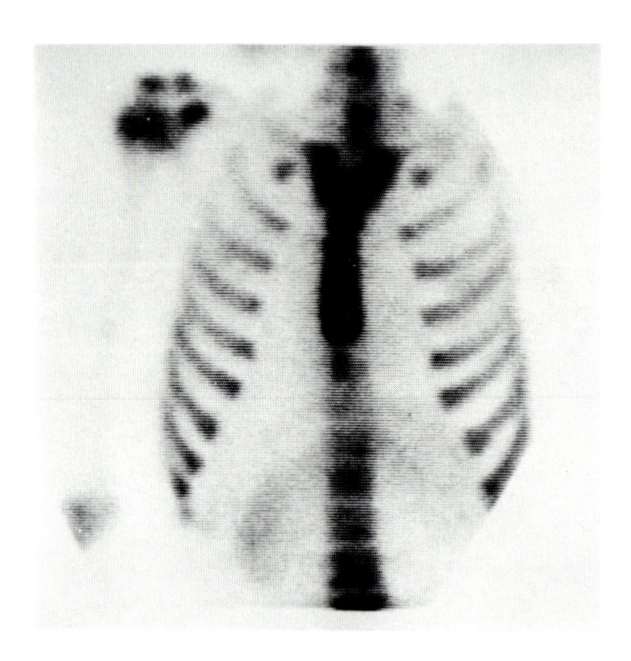

(i) The 11th and 12th ribs are posterior structures and are not visualised on this projection.

(ii) The bony portion of the 10th rib ends quite laterally and is usually not seen or, as in this illustration, may be faintly visible.

It will be appreciated from all the above images — but especially from the scintigram and photograph — just how extensive a cartilogenous portion of rib exists. In the photograph white represents rib, and black cartilage.

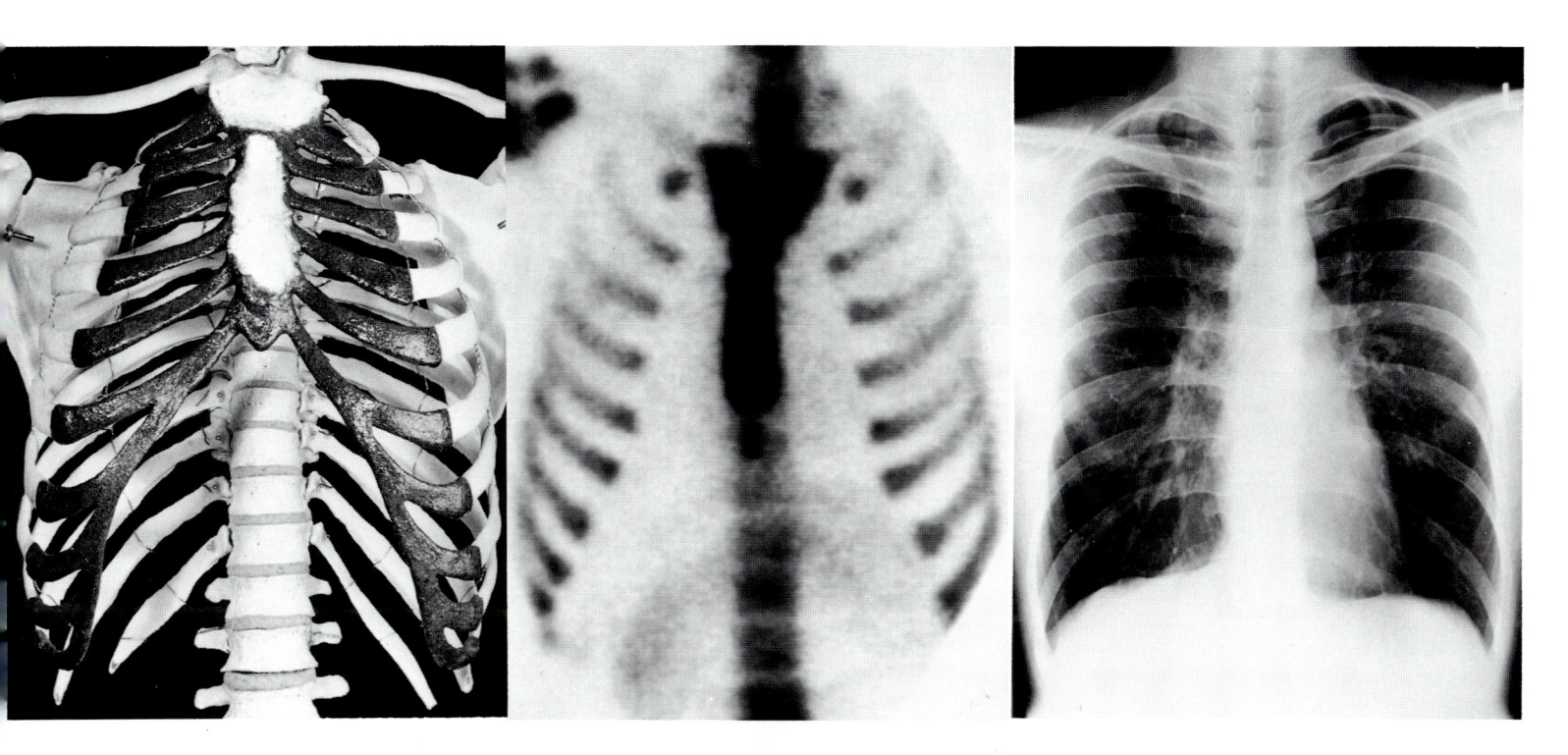

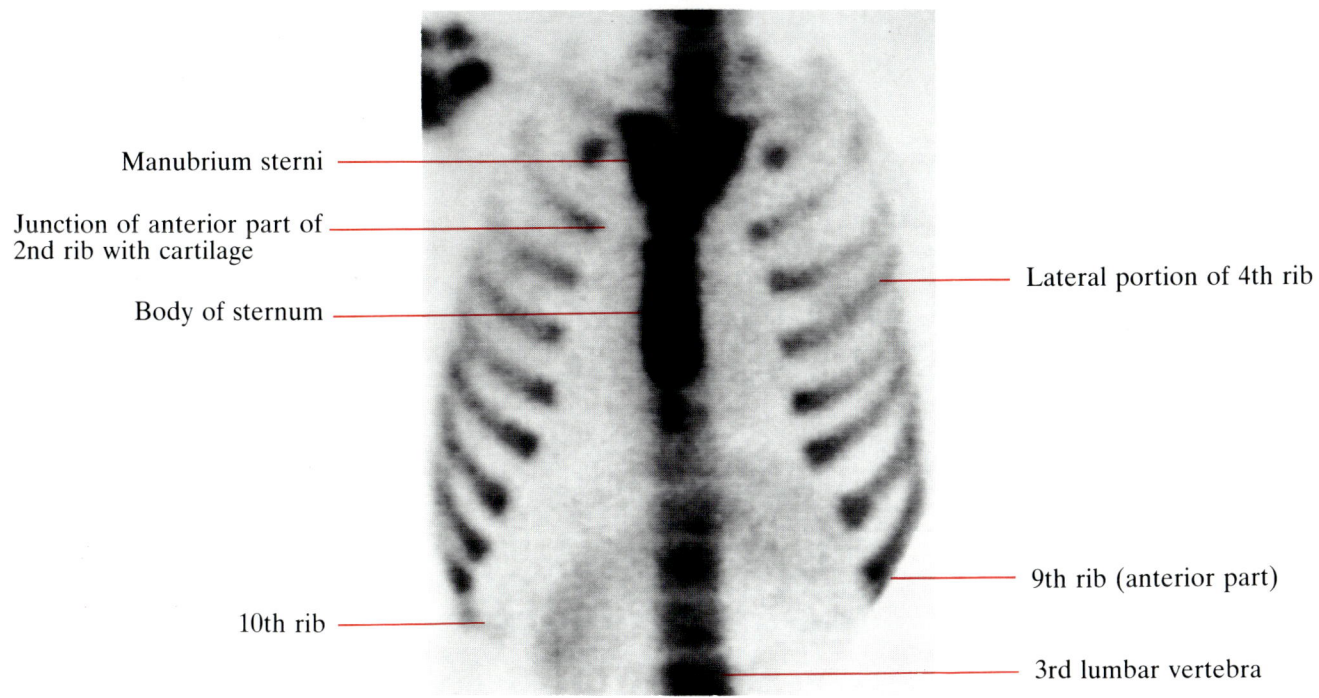

Manubrium sterni

Junction of anterior part of 2nd rib with cartilage

Body of sternum

10th rib

Lateral portion of 4th rib

9th rib (anterior part)

3rd lumbar vertebra

39

Posterior view of thoracic cage

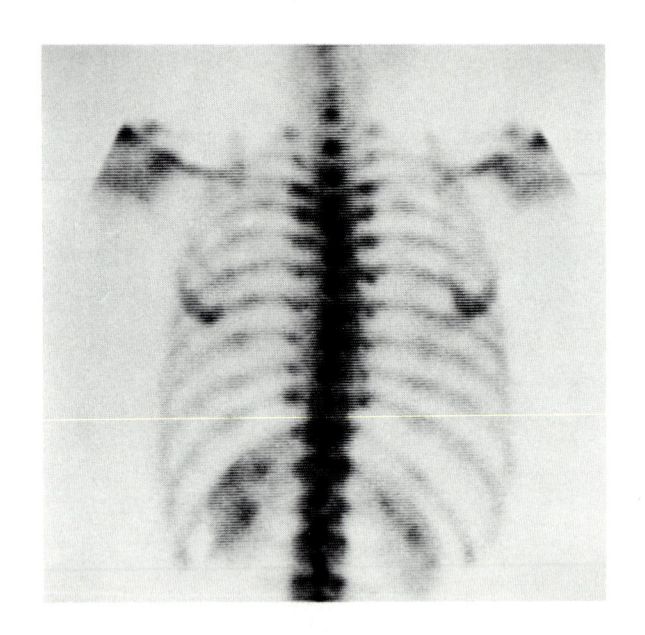

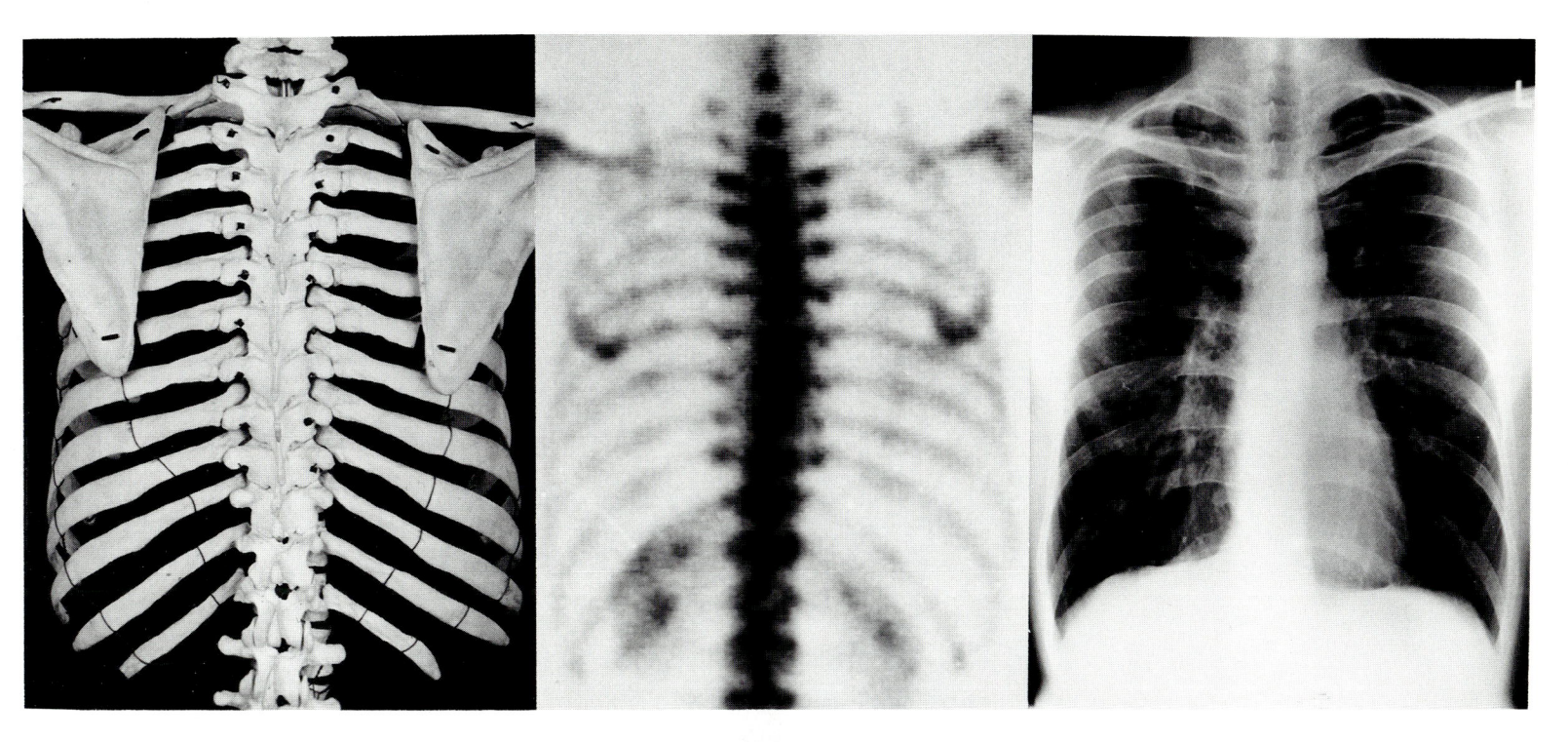

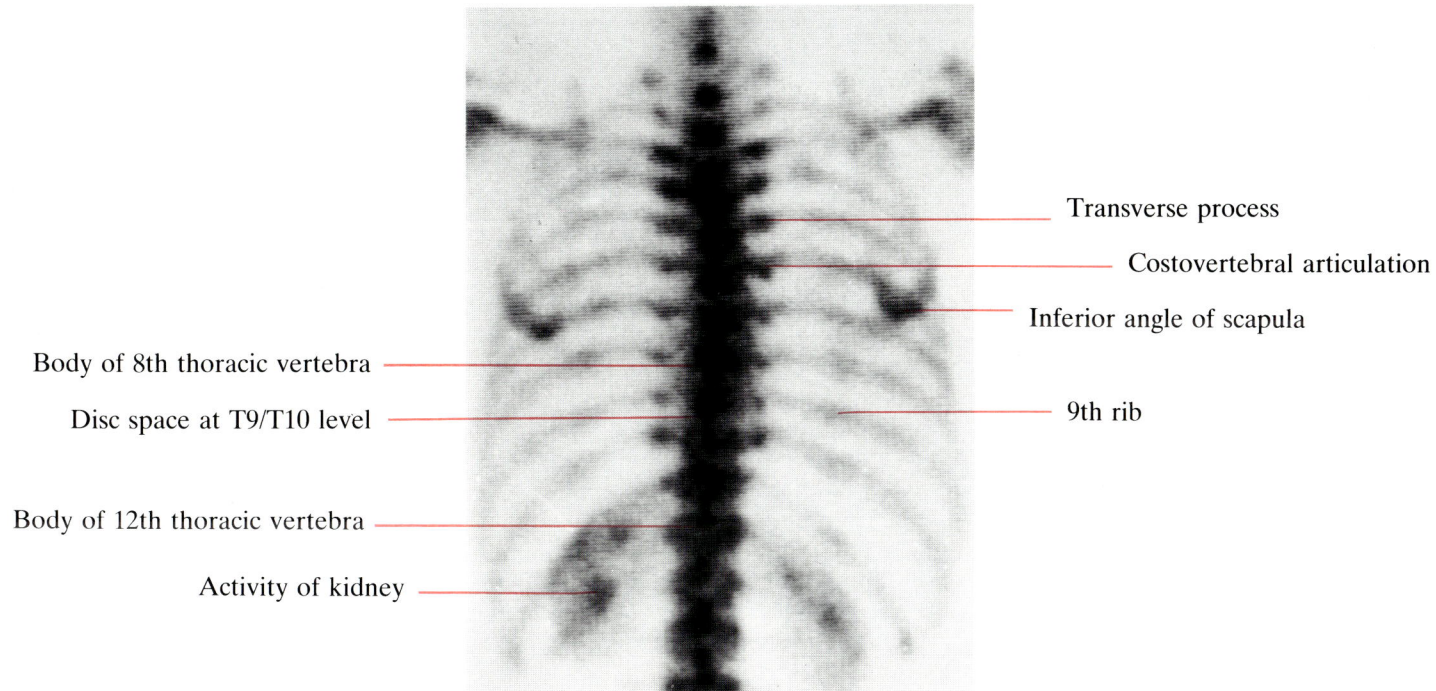

Transverse process
Costovertebral articulation
Inferior angle of scapula

Body of 8th thoracic vertebra
Disc space at T9/T10 level   9th rib

Body of 12th thoracic vertebra
Activity of kidney

41

Posterior view of thoracic spine

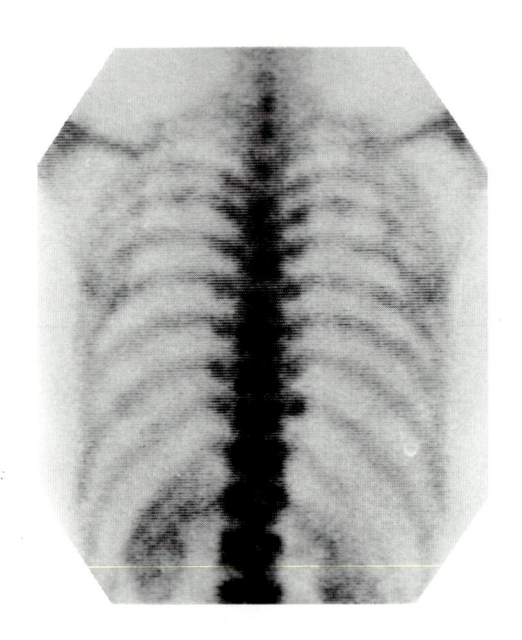

(i) The upper thoracic spine is seen (less well) as an area of decreased activity when imaging the whole thoracic column. This is an expected finding since the normal thoracic kyphosis places that part of the spine a little further from the camera.

(ii) Disc spaces always appear as areas of decreased activity in normal subjects.

Transverse process of T5

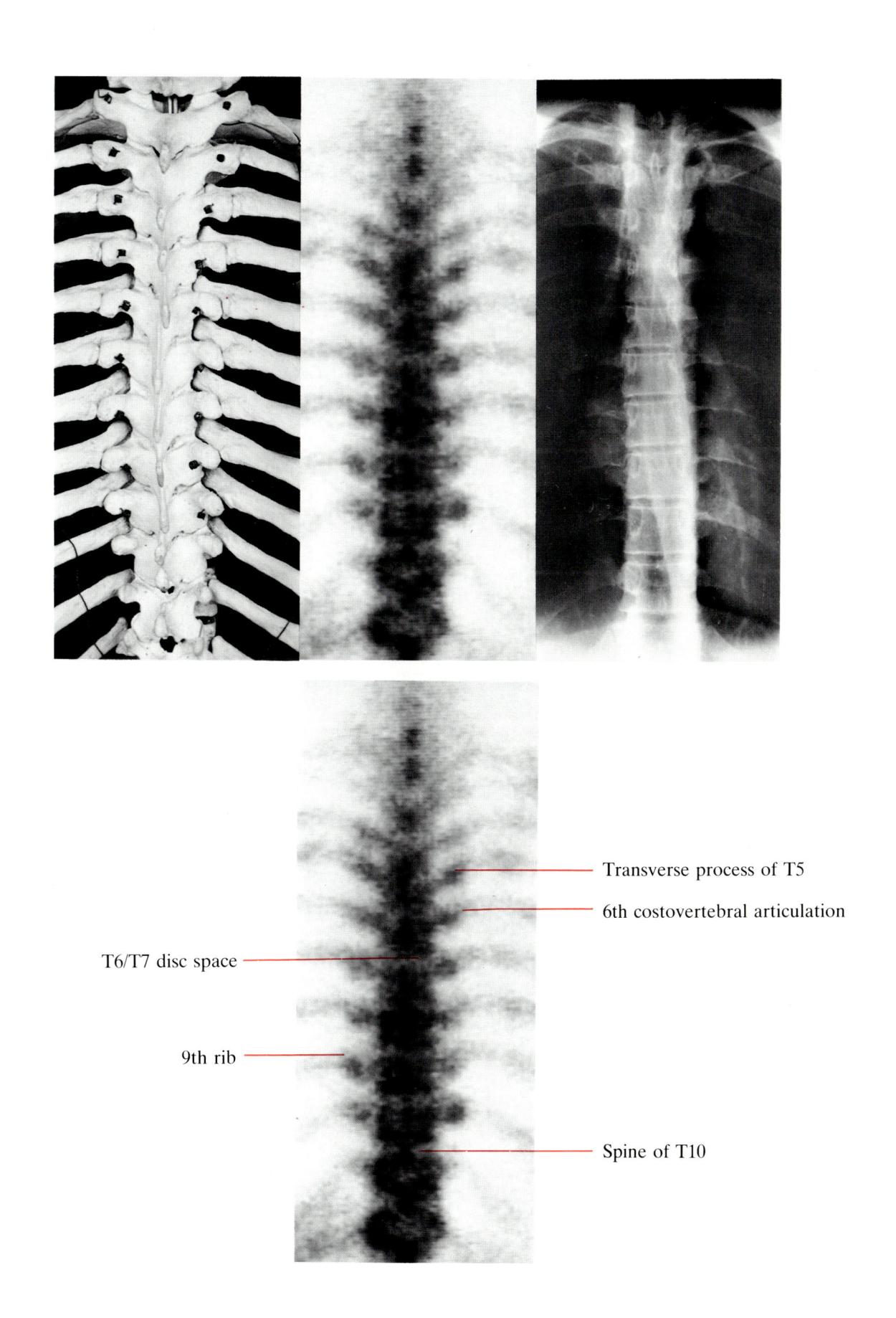

6th costovertebral articulation

T6/T7 disc space

9th rib

Spine of T10

Oblique lumbar spine

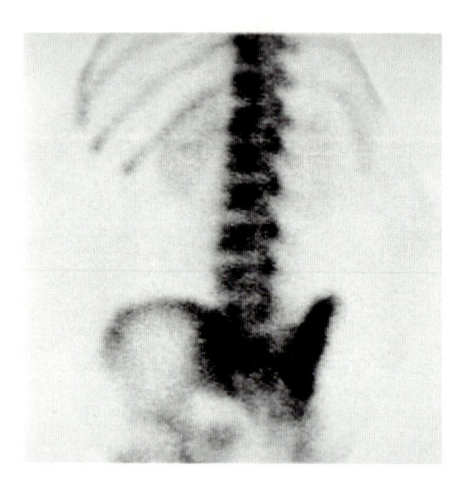

(i) The pars interarticularis is a thin bony structure and takes up little radionucleide and therefore appears as an area of decreased activity. In cases of spondylolisthesis or spondylolysis it may appear as an area of increased activity.

(ii) The right apophyseal joint is the one which is imaged on scintigraphy and radiography but on skeletal photography it is the left side which is imaged.

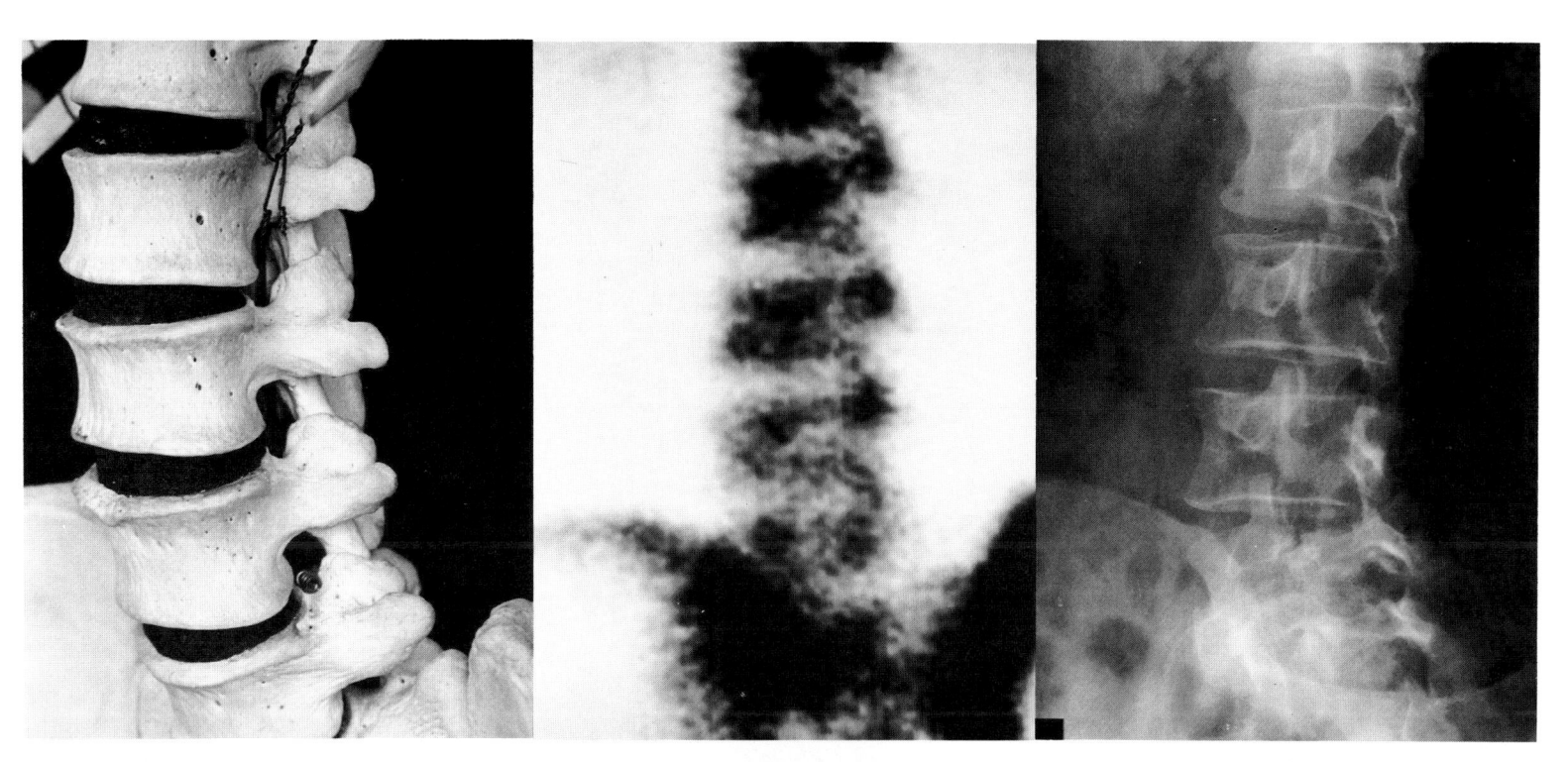

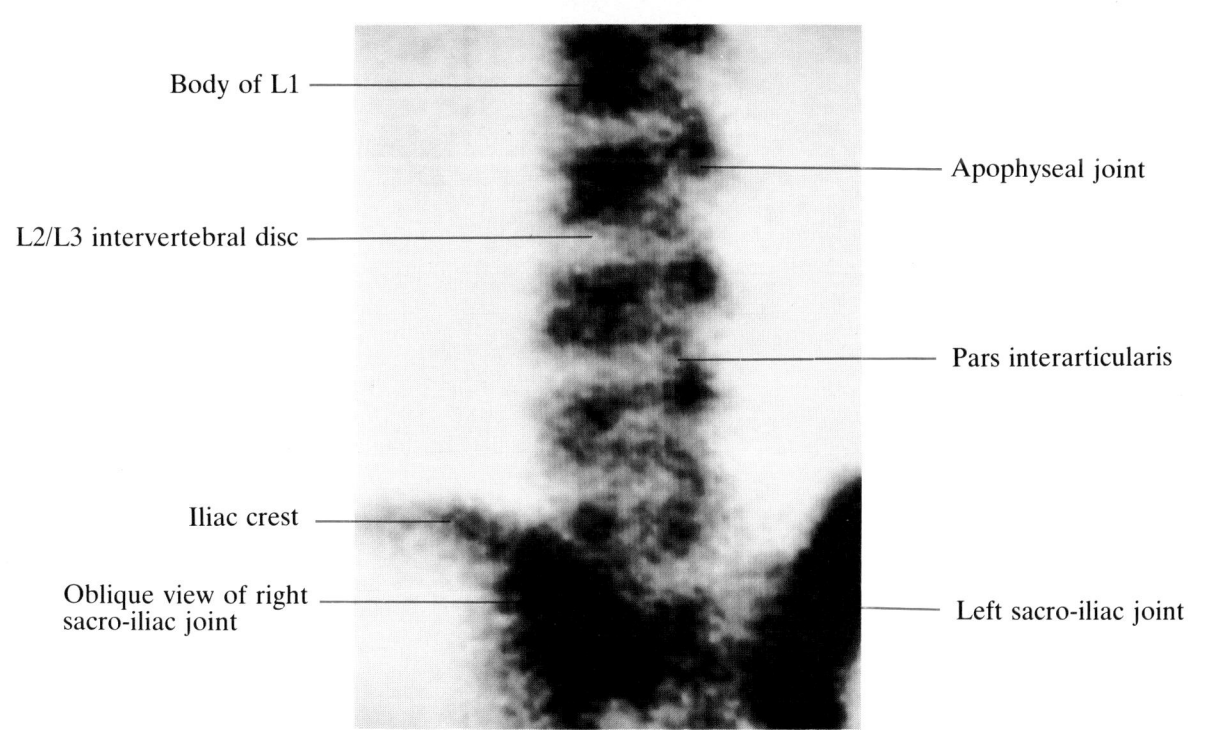

Body of L1

Apophyseal joint

L2/L3 intervertebral disc

Pars interarticularis

Iliac crest

Oblique view of right sacro-iliac joint

Left sacro-iliac joint

Posterior view of lumbar spine

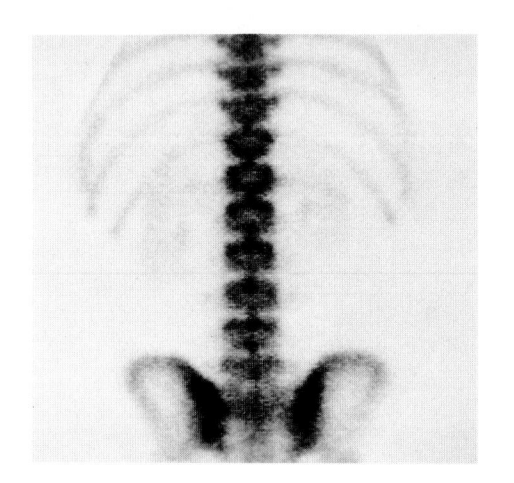

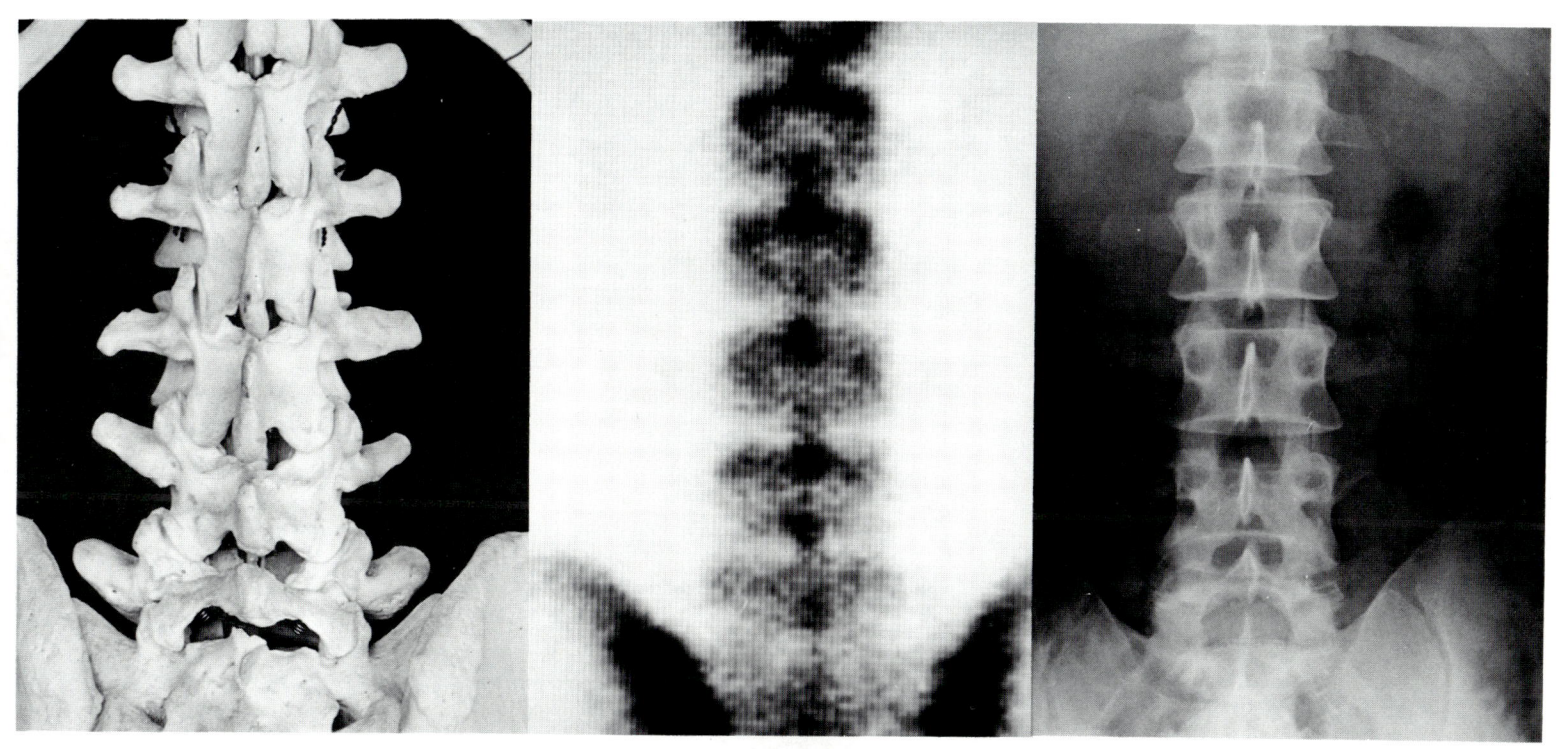

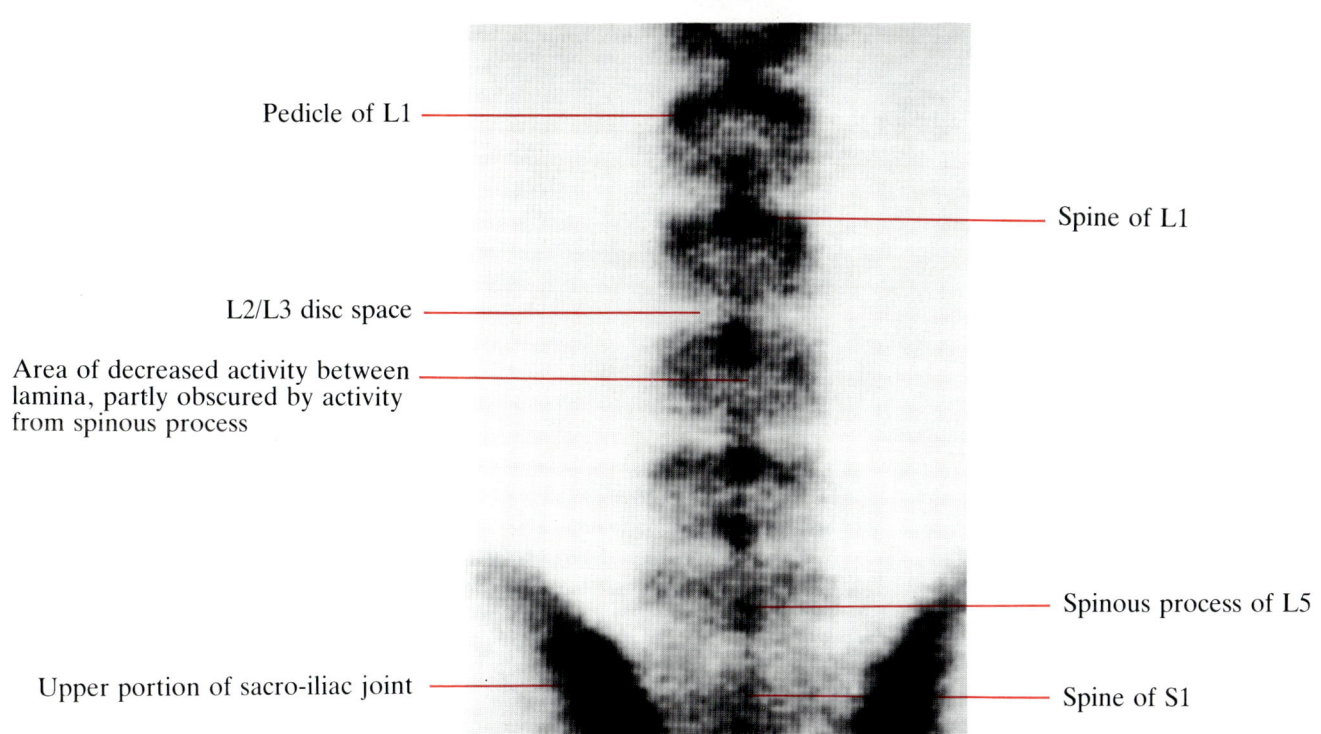

Pedicle of L1

Spine of L1

L2/L3 disc space

Area of decreased activity between lamina, partly obscured by activity from spinous process

Spinous process of L5

Upper portion of sacro-iliac joint

Spine of S1

Anterior view of pelvis

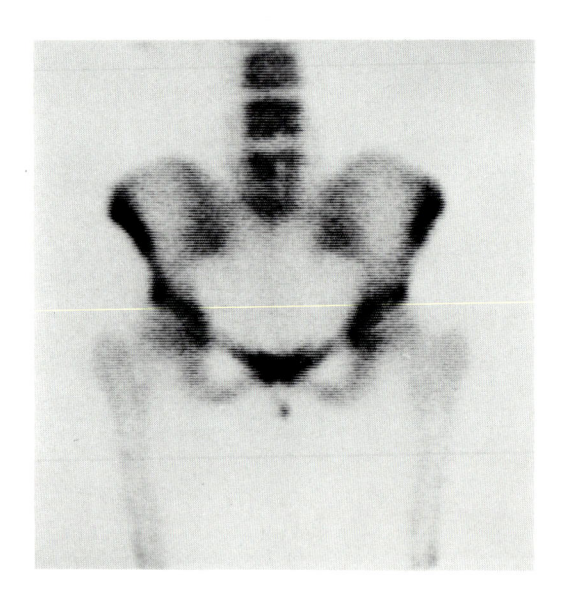

(i) The sacro-iliac joints and ischial tuberosities appear relatively inactive — an expected finding in this anterior view.

(ii) The area of increased activity just below the symphysis pubis is due to incontinence of radioactive urine, a not uncommon finding.

Anterior superior iliac spine

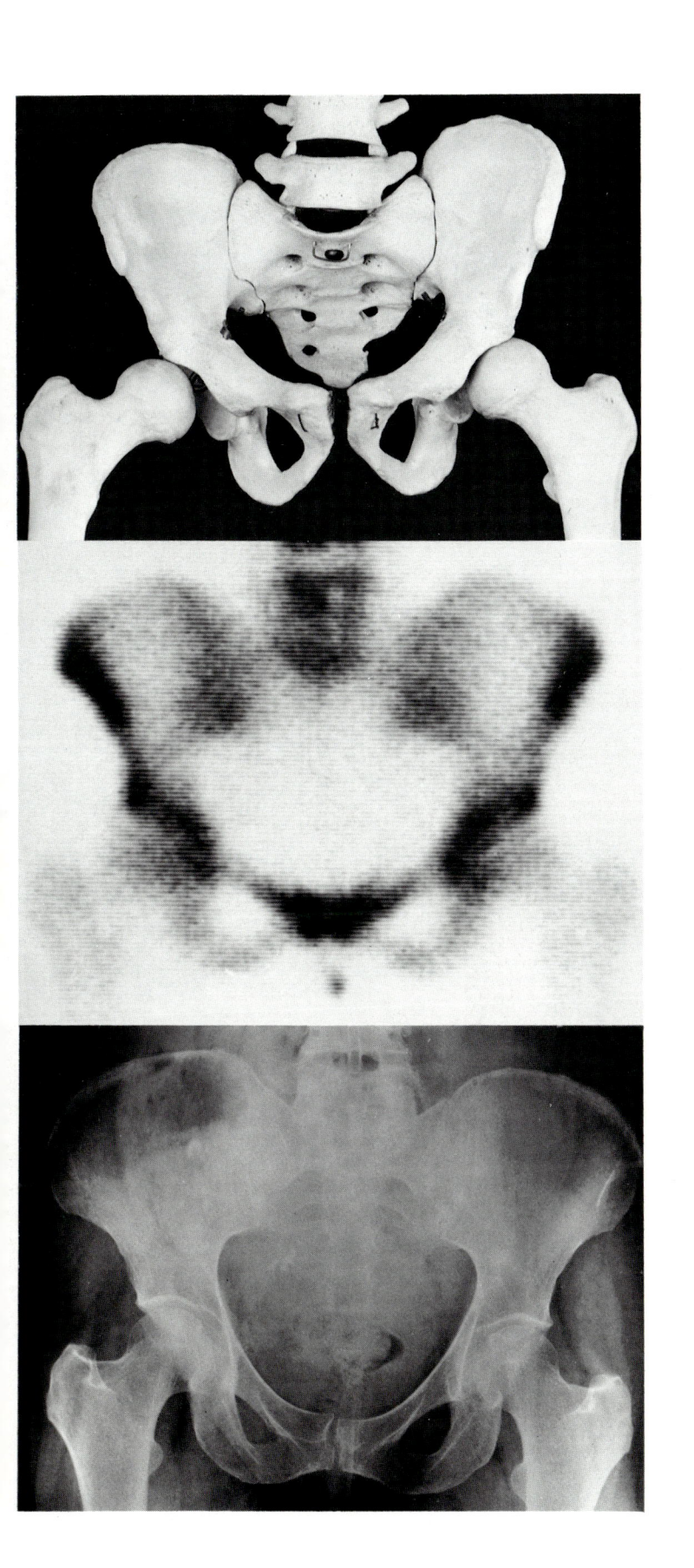

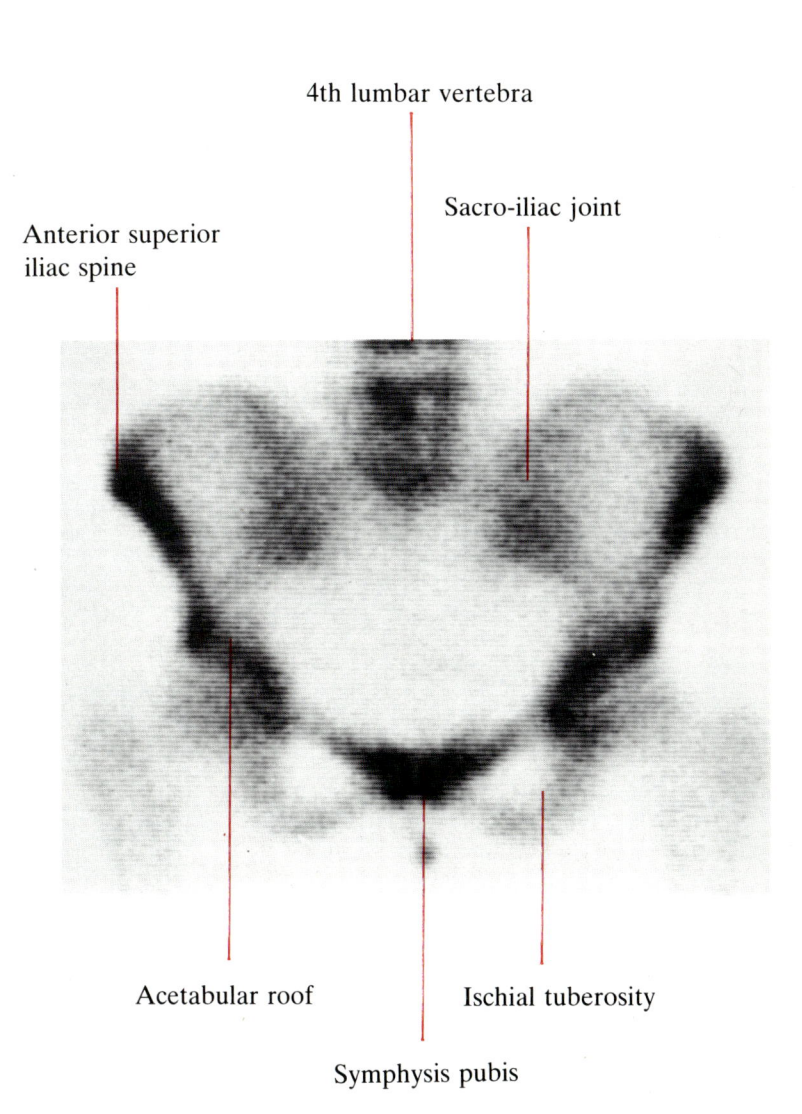

4th lumbar vertebra

Sacro-iliac joint

Acetabular roof

Ischial tuberosity

Symphysis pubis

Posterior view of pelvis

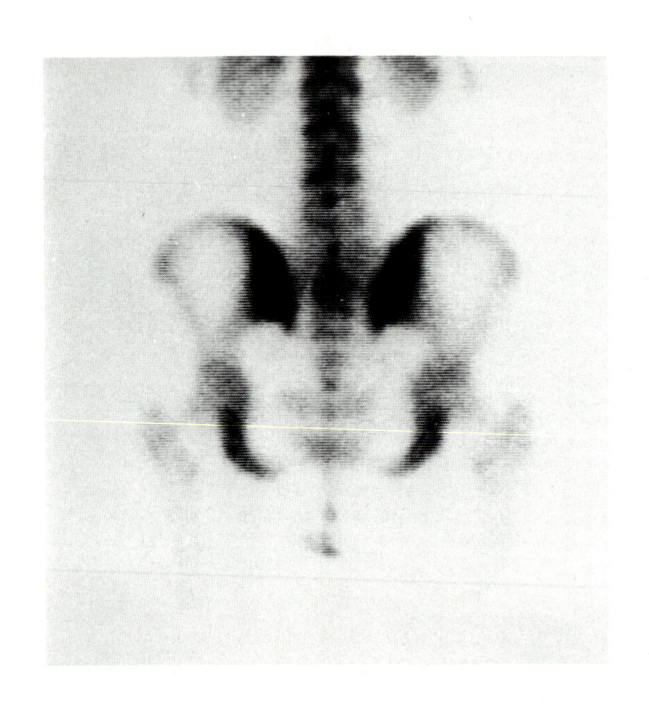

Left sacro-iliac joint

Sciatic foramen

L4

Iliac crest

Ischial tuberosity

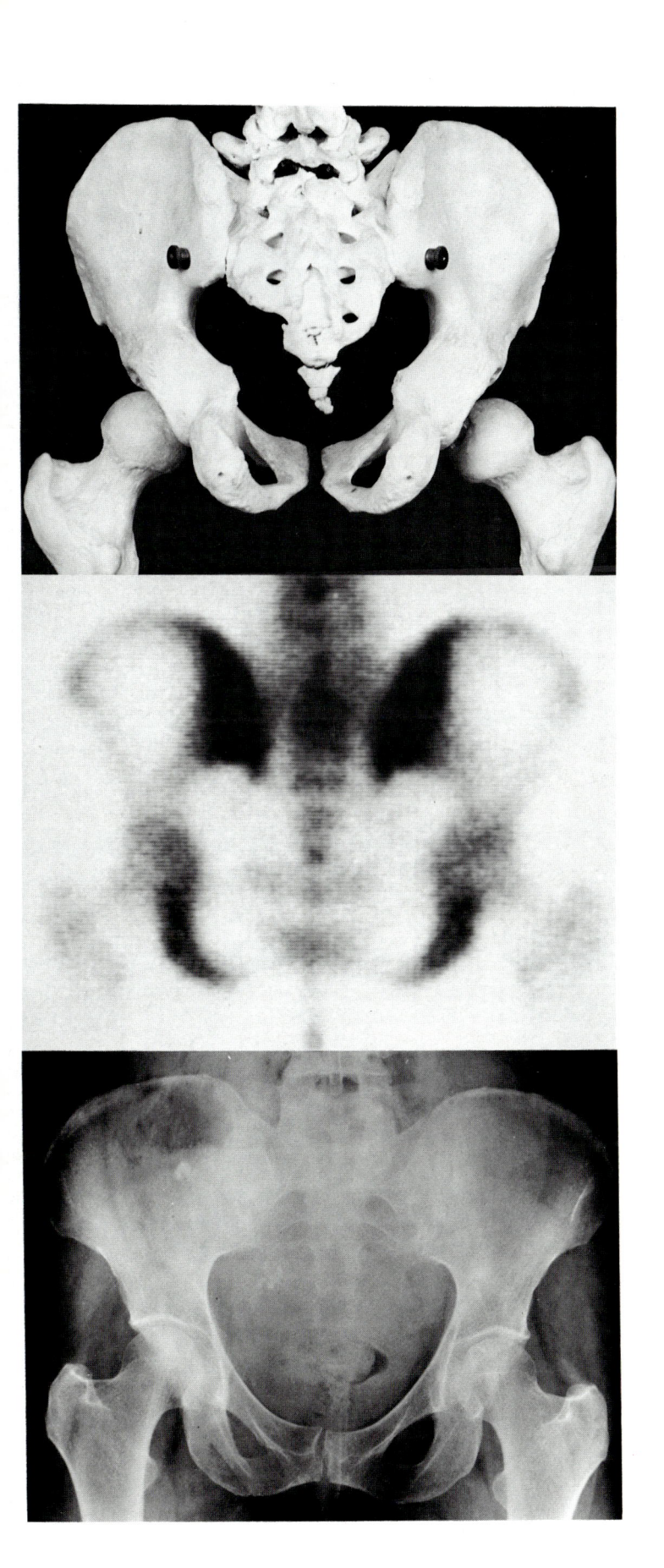

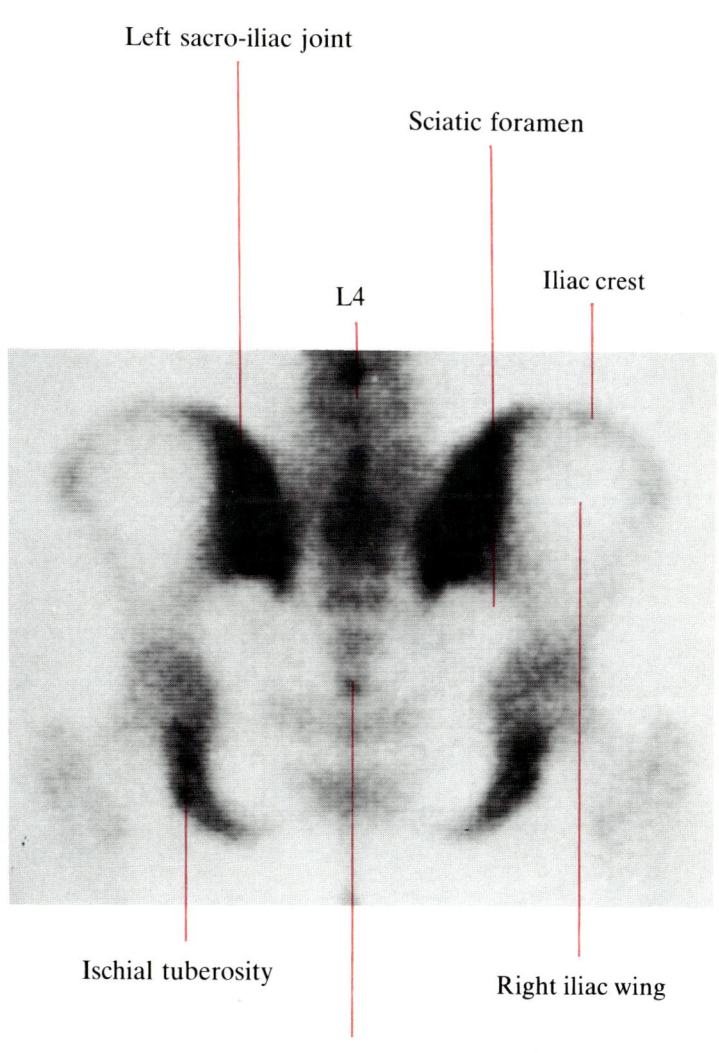

Right iliac wing

Lower sacral or upper coccygeal Vertebrae

51

Sacro-iliac joints

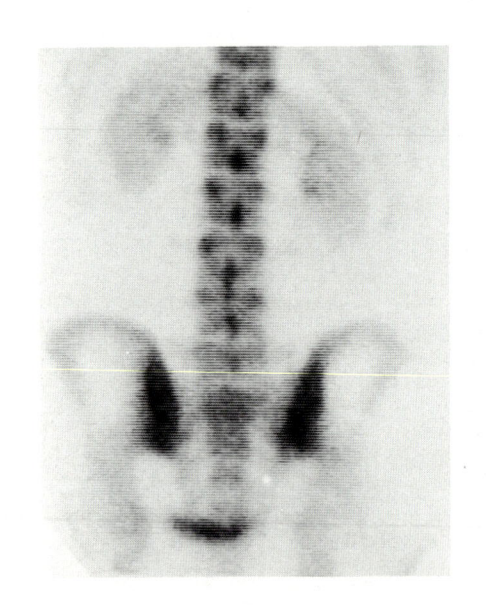

Spine of L5

Left sacro-iliac joint   Ala of sacrum

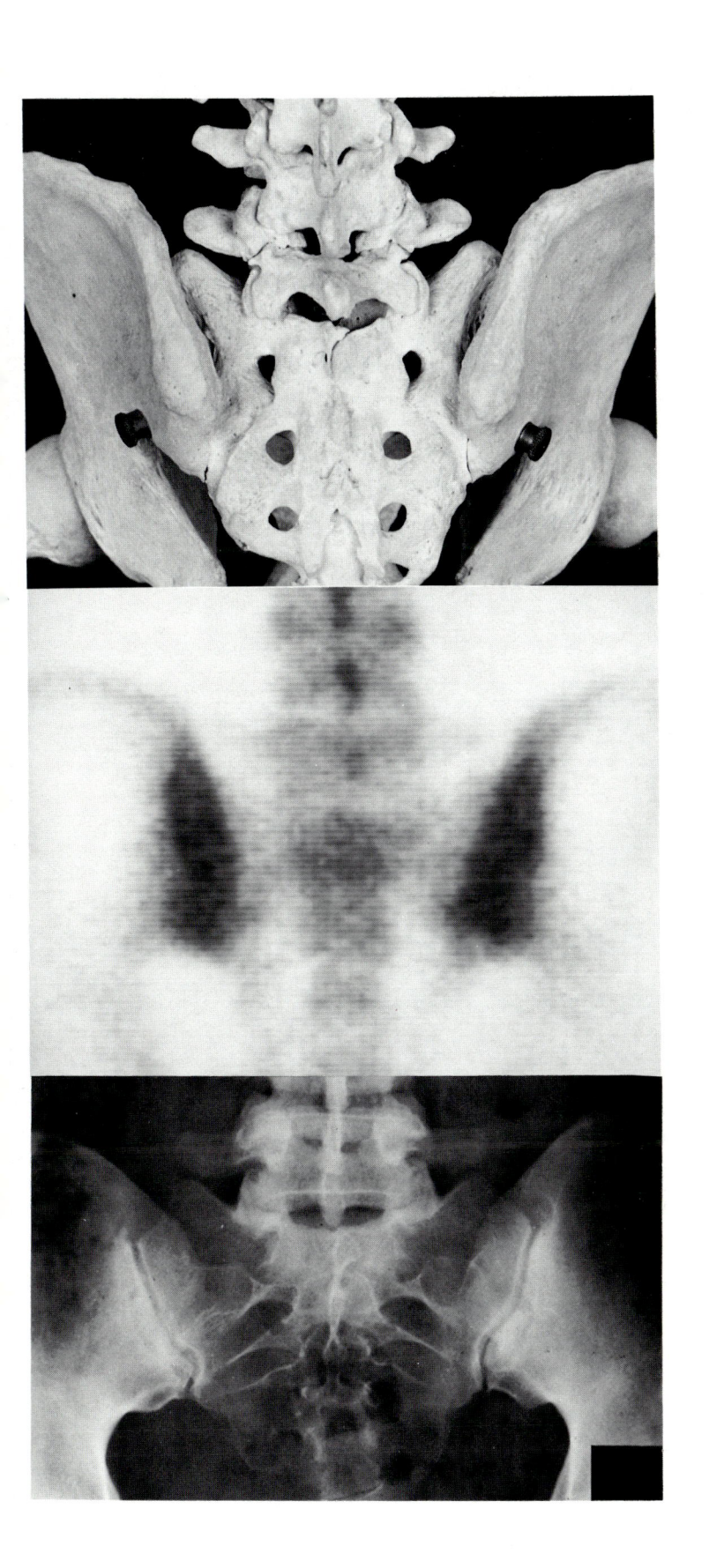

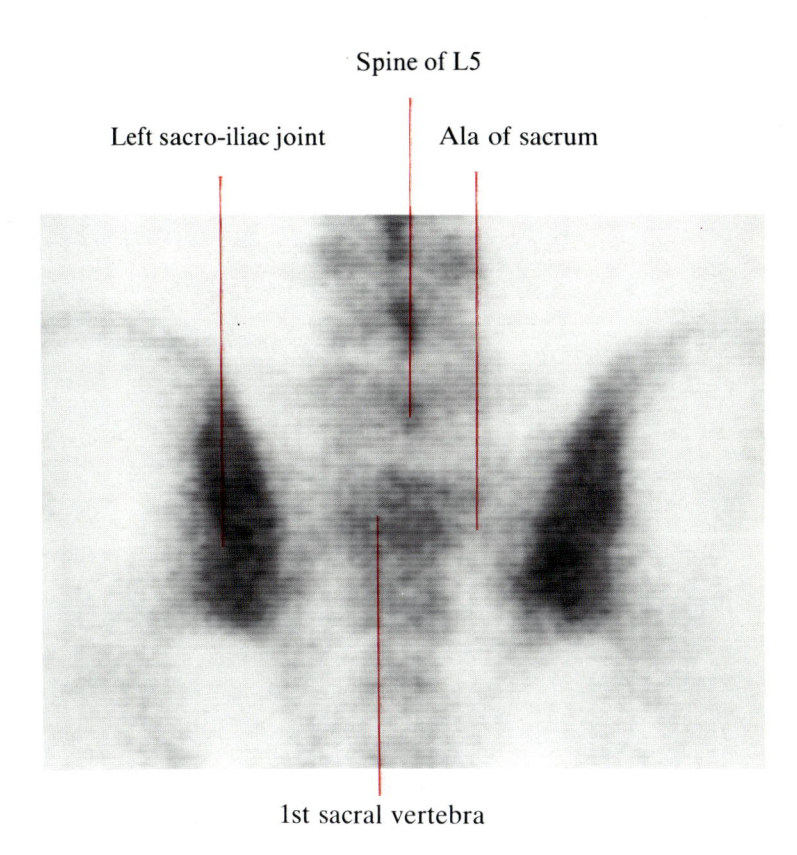

1st sacral vertebra

Posterior view of sacrum

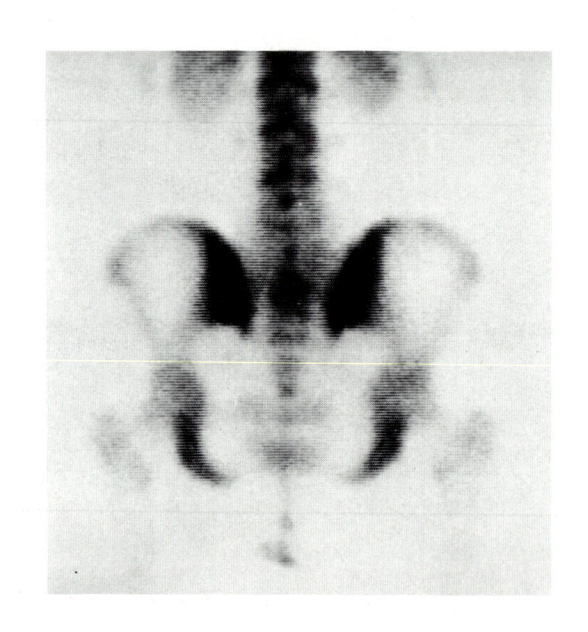

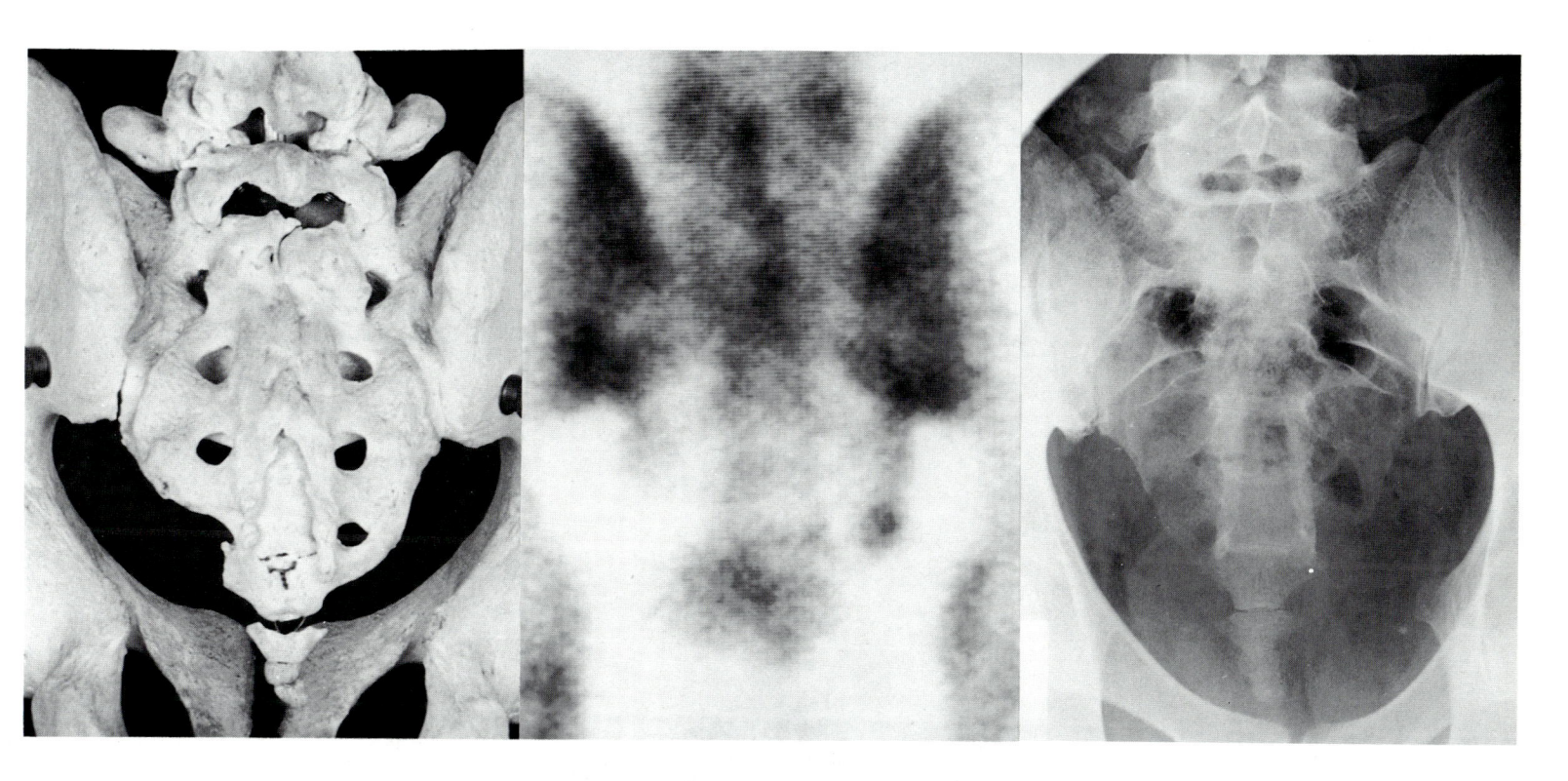

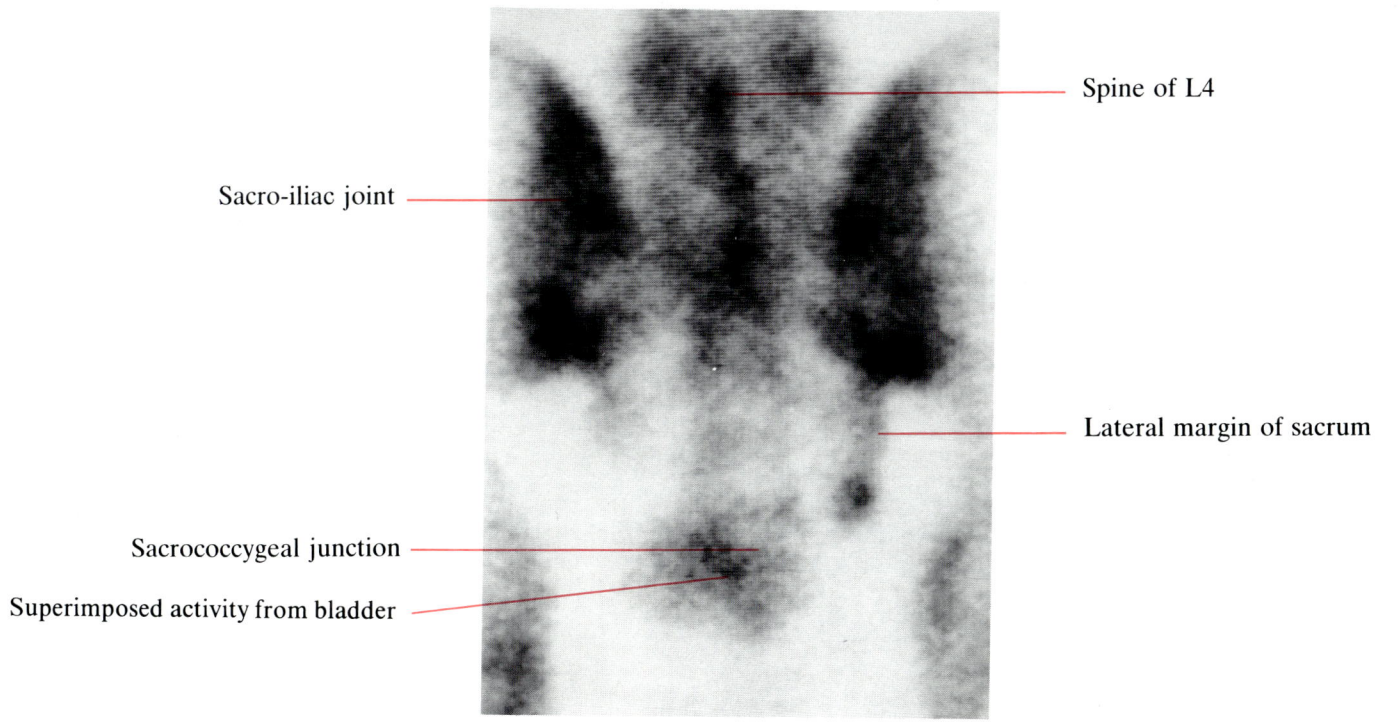

Spine of L4

Sacro-iliac joint

Lateral margin of sacrum

Sacrococcygeal junction
Superimposed activity from bladder

Posterior view of hip

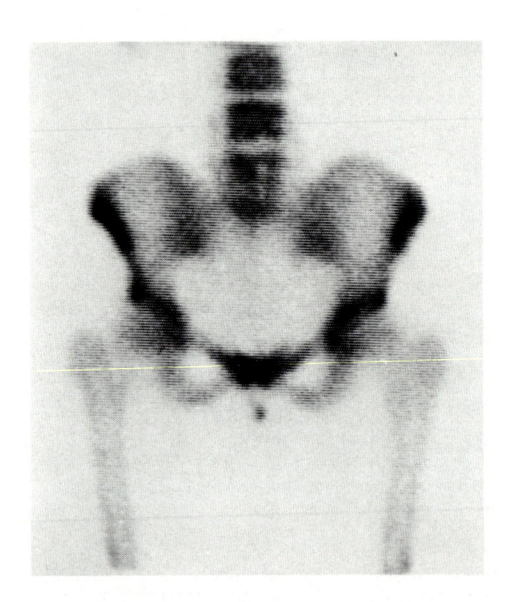

(i) The area of increased activity above the superior pubic ramus within the pelvis represents the bladder. This is a normal finding in bone scintigraphy since the isotope is excreted by the kidneys.

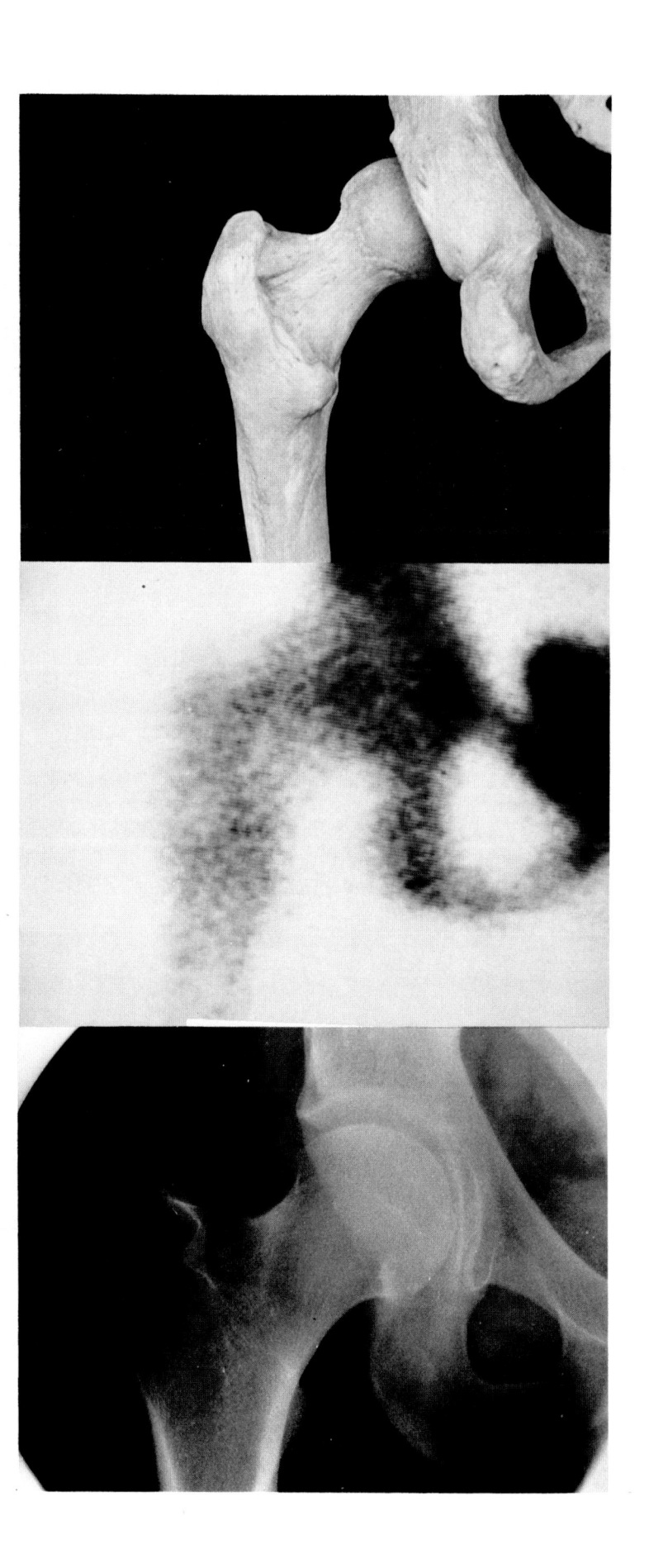

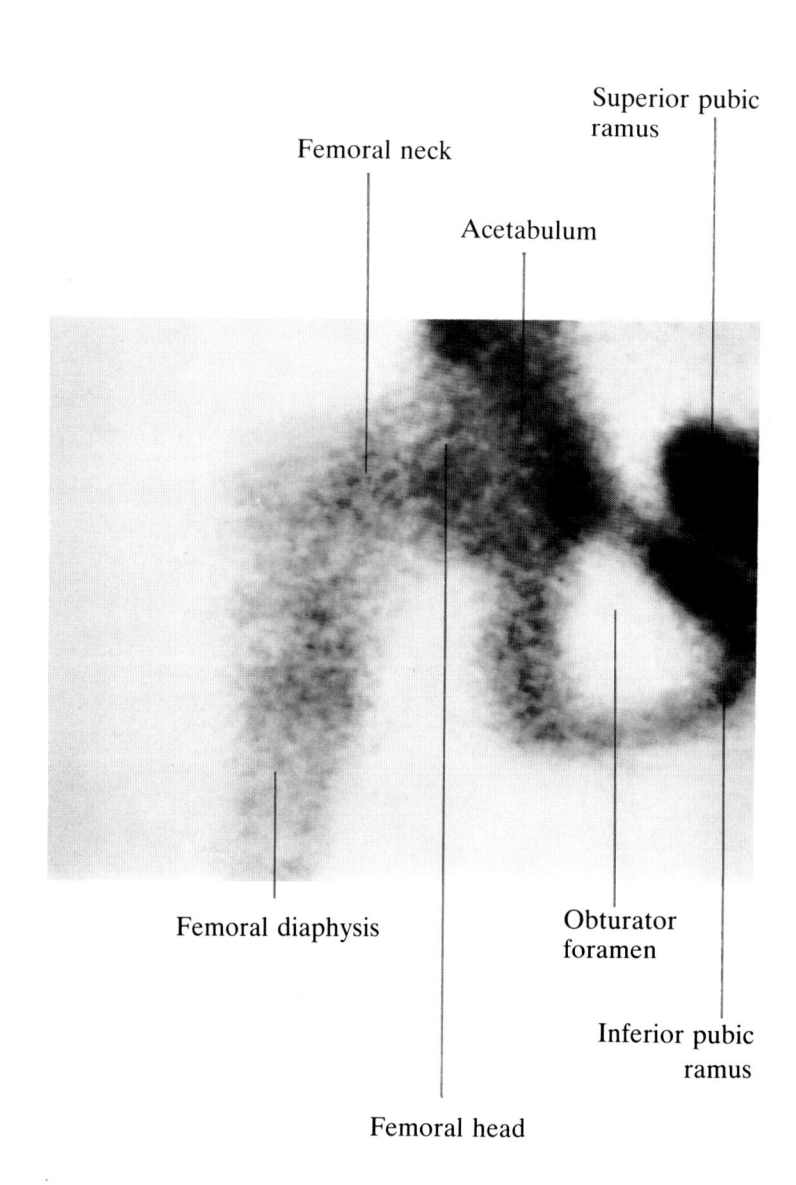

Femoral neck
Superior pubic ramus
Acetabulum
Femoral diaphysis
Obturator foramen
Inferior pubic ramus
Femoral head

Anterior view of femur

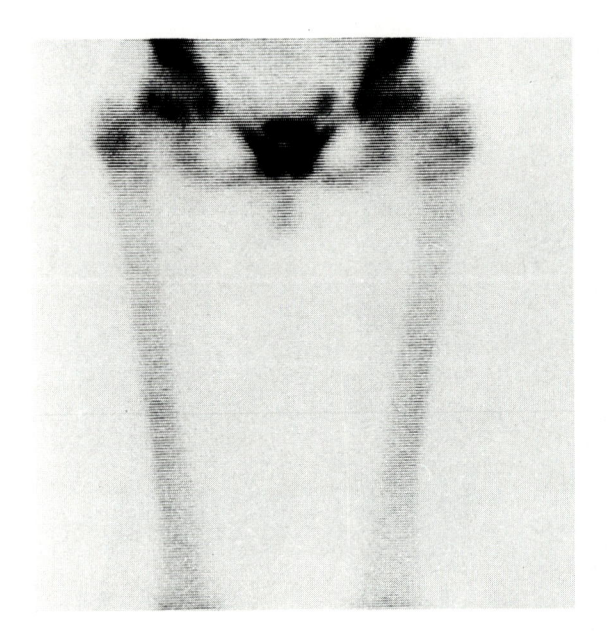

(i) An area of increased activity is seen in the region of the intertrochanteric line of the scintigram. This is due to the pull exerted by the quadratus femorus, gluteous medius and a variety of ligaments which are attached here, often causing excitation of bone (as in this case) and resultant increased activity. Occasionally increased activity is seen over the lesser trochanter for the same reason except this time the ilio psoas is the muscle involved. In many people, however, the lesser trochanter is often only barely visible as illustrated here.

(ii) The articular portion of the lower femur is marginally off the scintigram and the tibial plateaus have not been included.

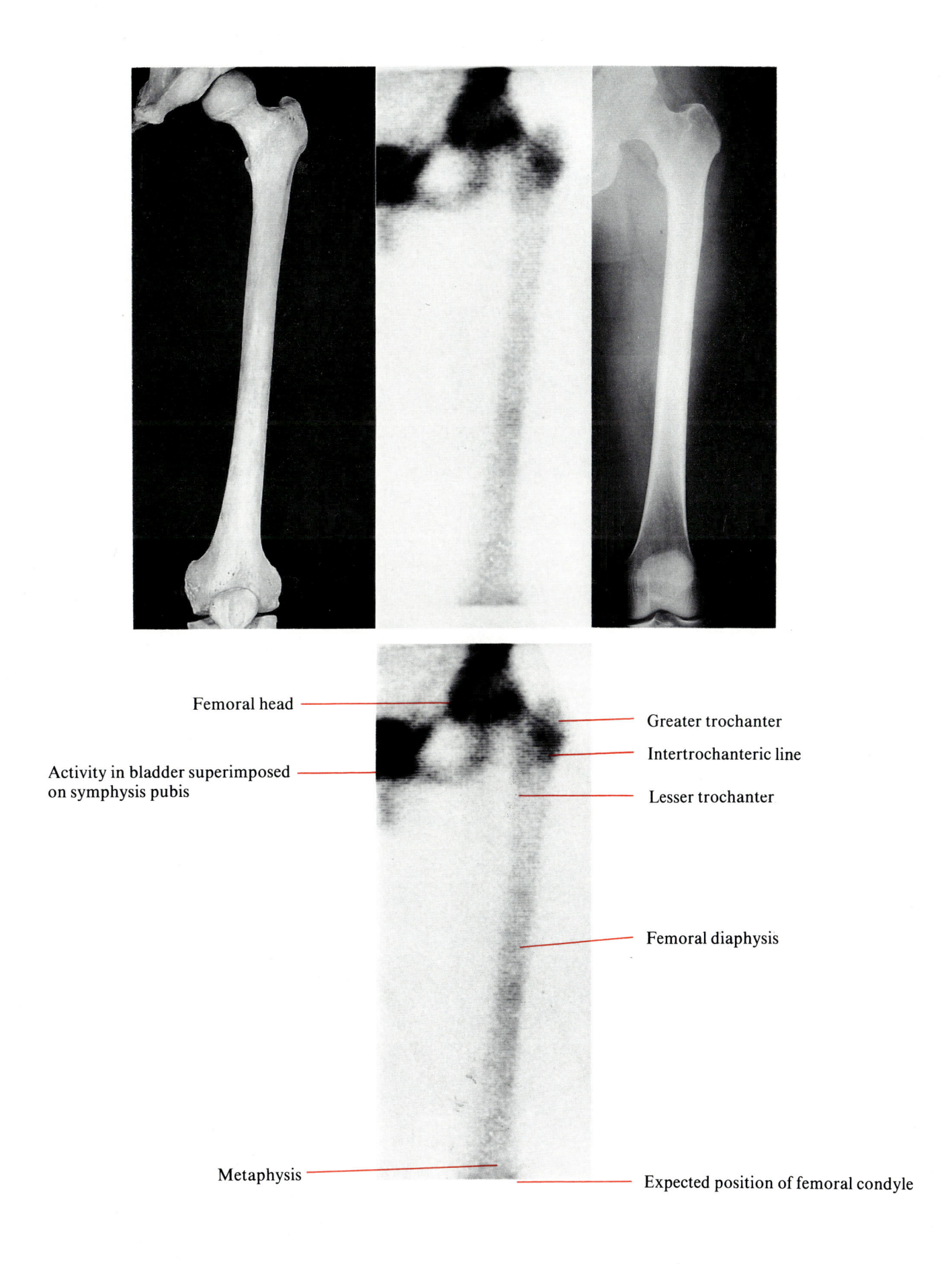

Femoral head — Greater trochanter
 — Intertrochanteric line
Activity in bladder superimposed on symphysis pubis — Lesser trochanter

Femoral diaphysis

Metaphysis — Expected position of femoral condyle

59

Lateral view of knee

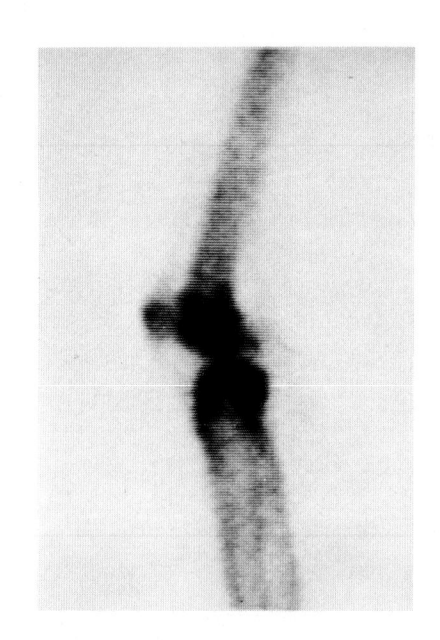

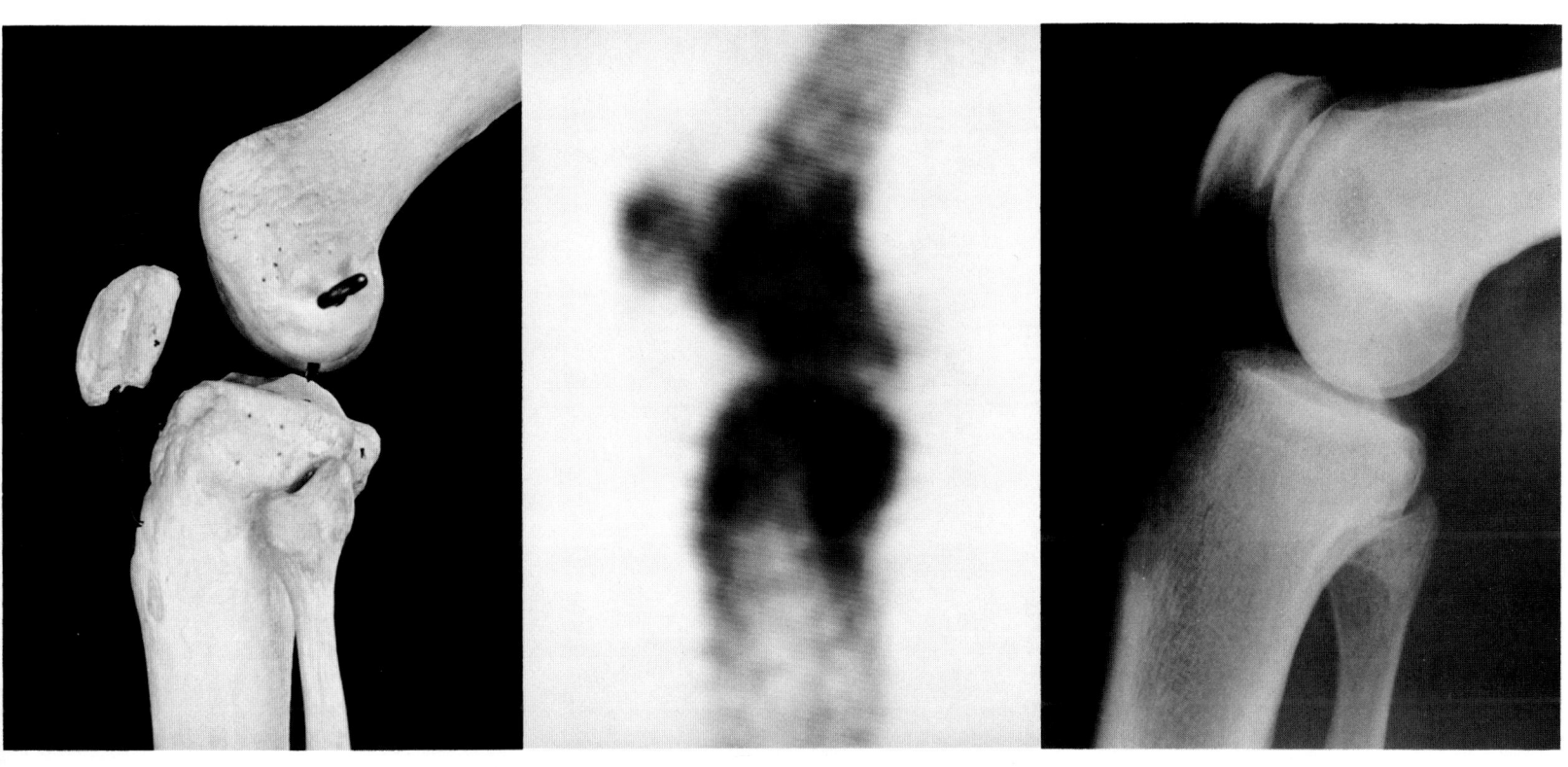

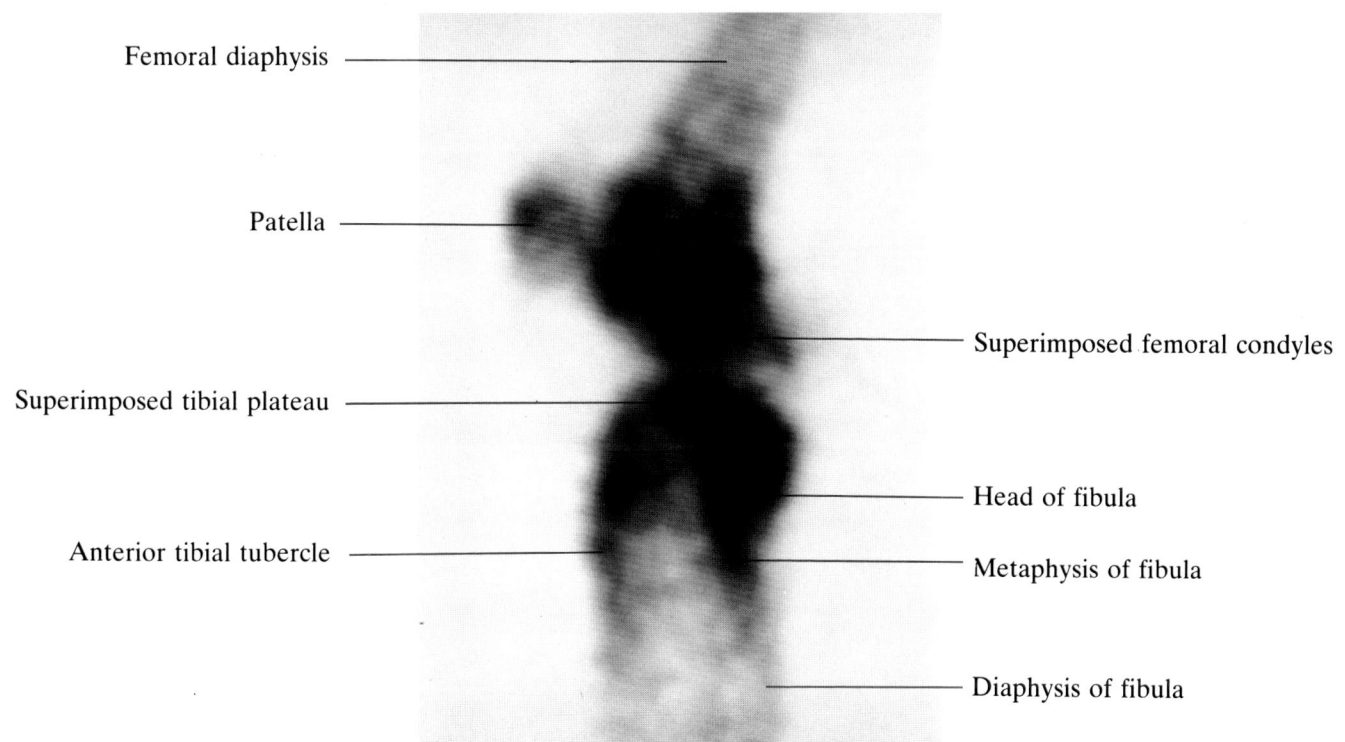

Femoral diaphysis

Patella

Superimposed tibial plateau

Anterior tibial tubercle

Superimposed femoral condyles

Head of fibula

Metaphysis of fibula

Diaphysis of fibula

61

Posterior view of knee

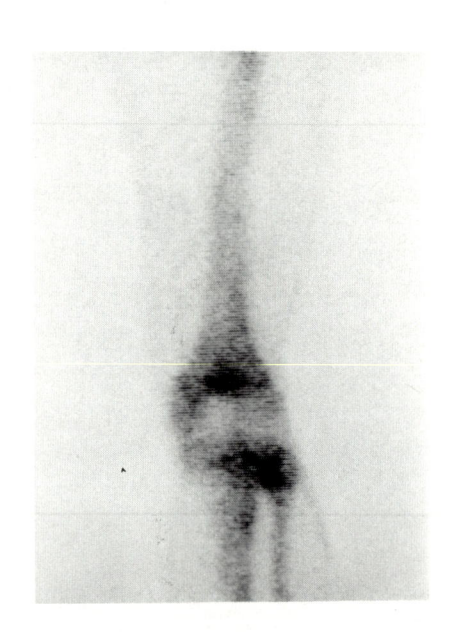

Femoral diaphysis

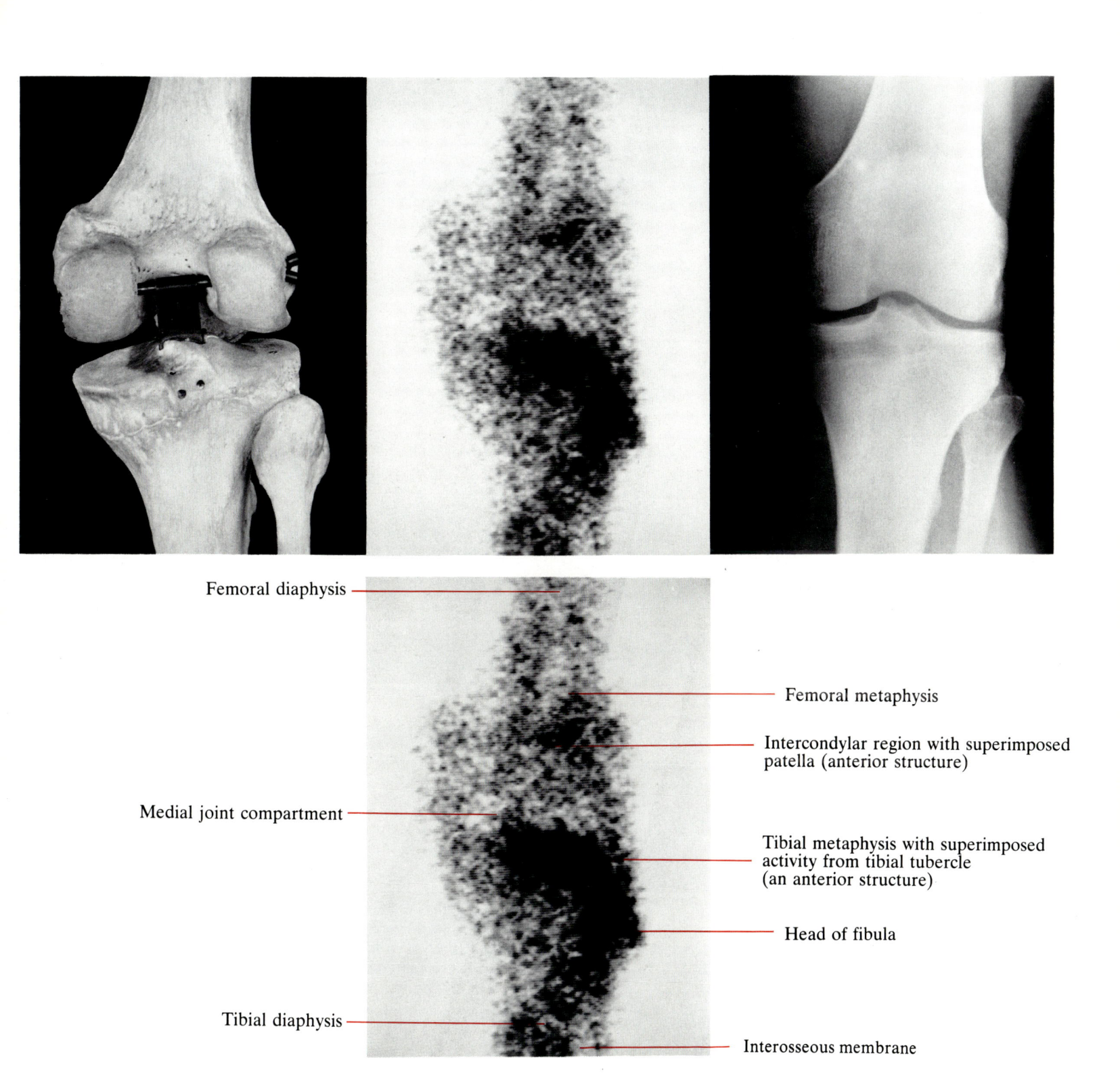

Femoral metaphysis

Intercondylar region with superimposed patella (anterior structure)

Medial joint compartment

Tibial metaphysis with superimposed activity from tibial tubercle (an anterior structure)

Head of fibula

Tibial diaphysis

Interosseous membrane

Anterior view of tibia and fibula

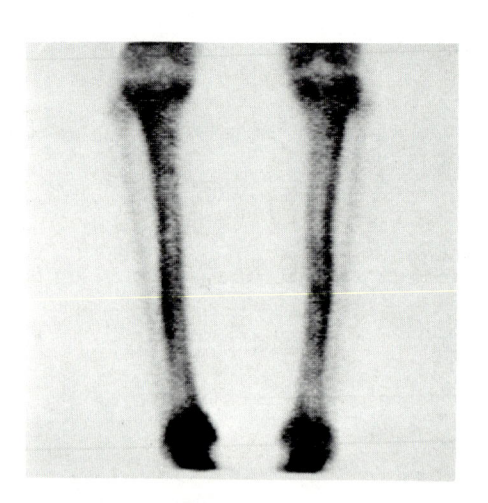

(i) As expected the thin bony structure of the fibula is reflected by its decrease in tracer activity and resultant poor image. Nevertheless we can visualise almost the entire structure.

(ii) The uneven distribution of tracer activity in the tibia is related to tendinous origins and insertions at which points activity is greatest.

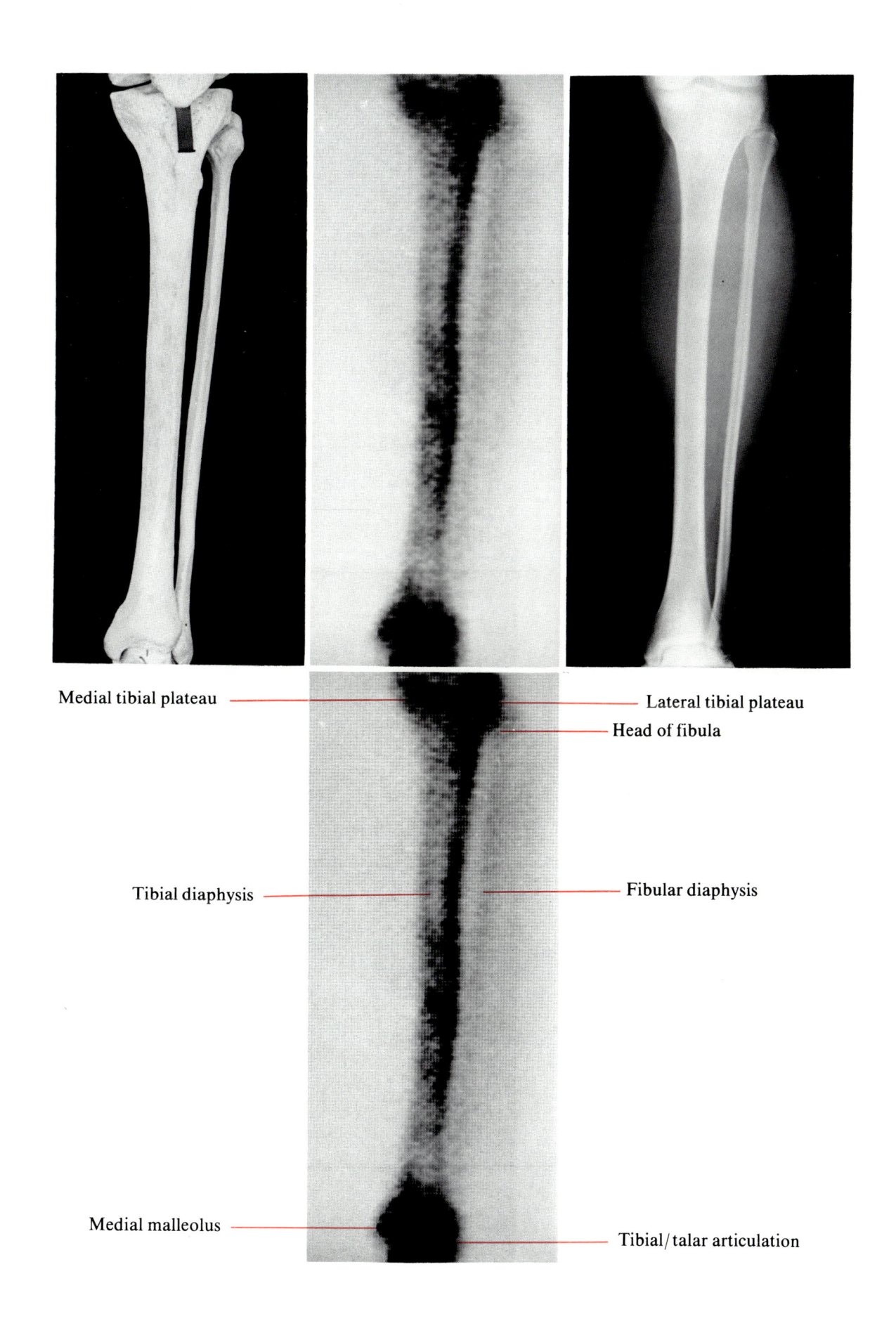

Medial tibial plateau —————— ————— Lateral tibial plateau
————— Head of fibula

Tibial diaphysis —————— ————— Fibular diaphysis

Medial malleolus —————— ————— Tibial/talar articulation

Ankle

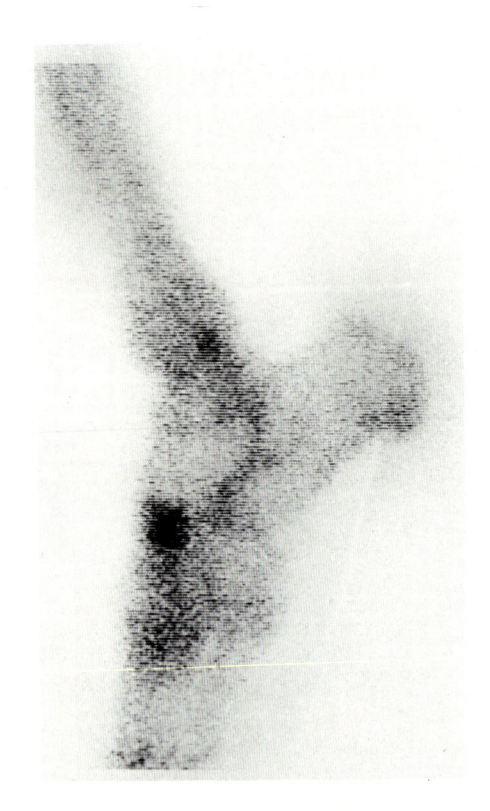

(i) Both the fibula and tibia are seen since this is not a perfect lateral view.

(ii) The medial cuneiform and first metatarsal are only seen in their entirety on the scintigram.

Fibula

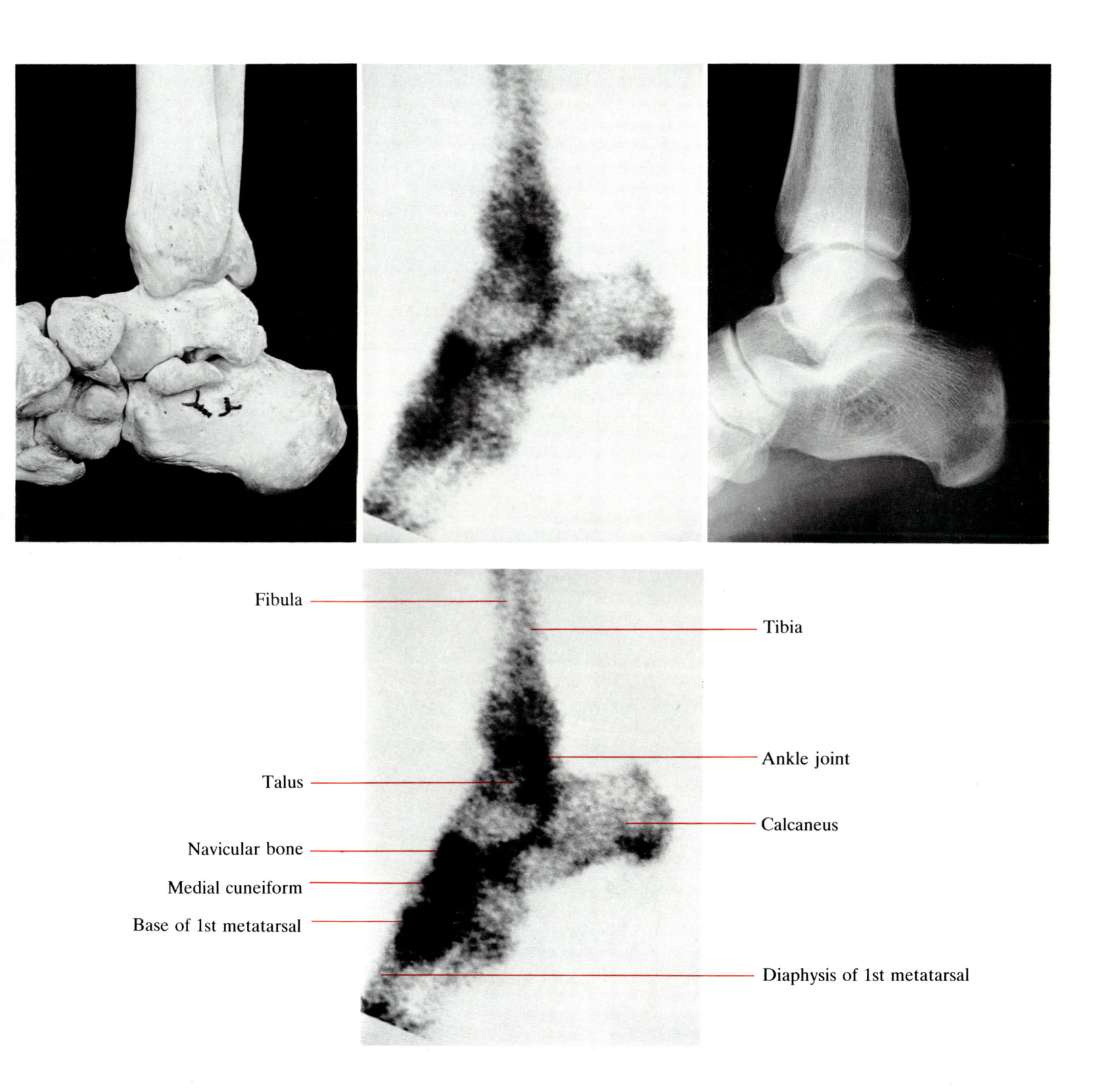

Tibia

Talus

Ankle joint

Navicular bone

Calcaneus

Medial cuneiform

Base of 1st metatarsal

Diaphysis of 1st metatarsal

67

Foot

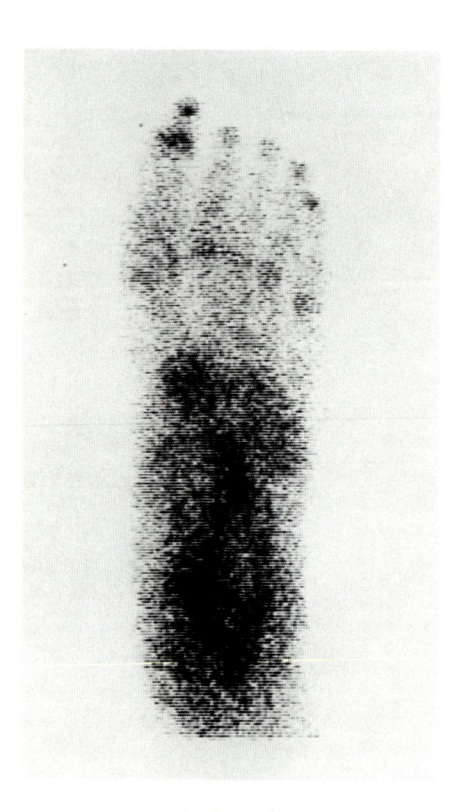

(i) The joints of the tarsus and long bones of the foot appear as areas of increased activity in normal patients who are asymptomatic and have normal radiographs.

(ii) In normal elderly patients individual metacarpo-phalangeal and interphalangeal joints may appear as areas of increased activity.

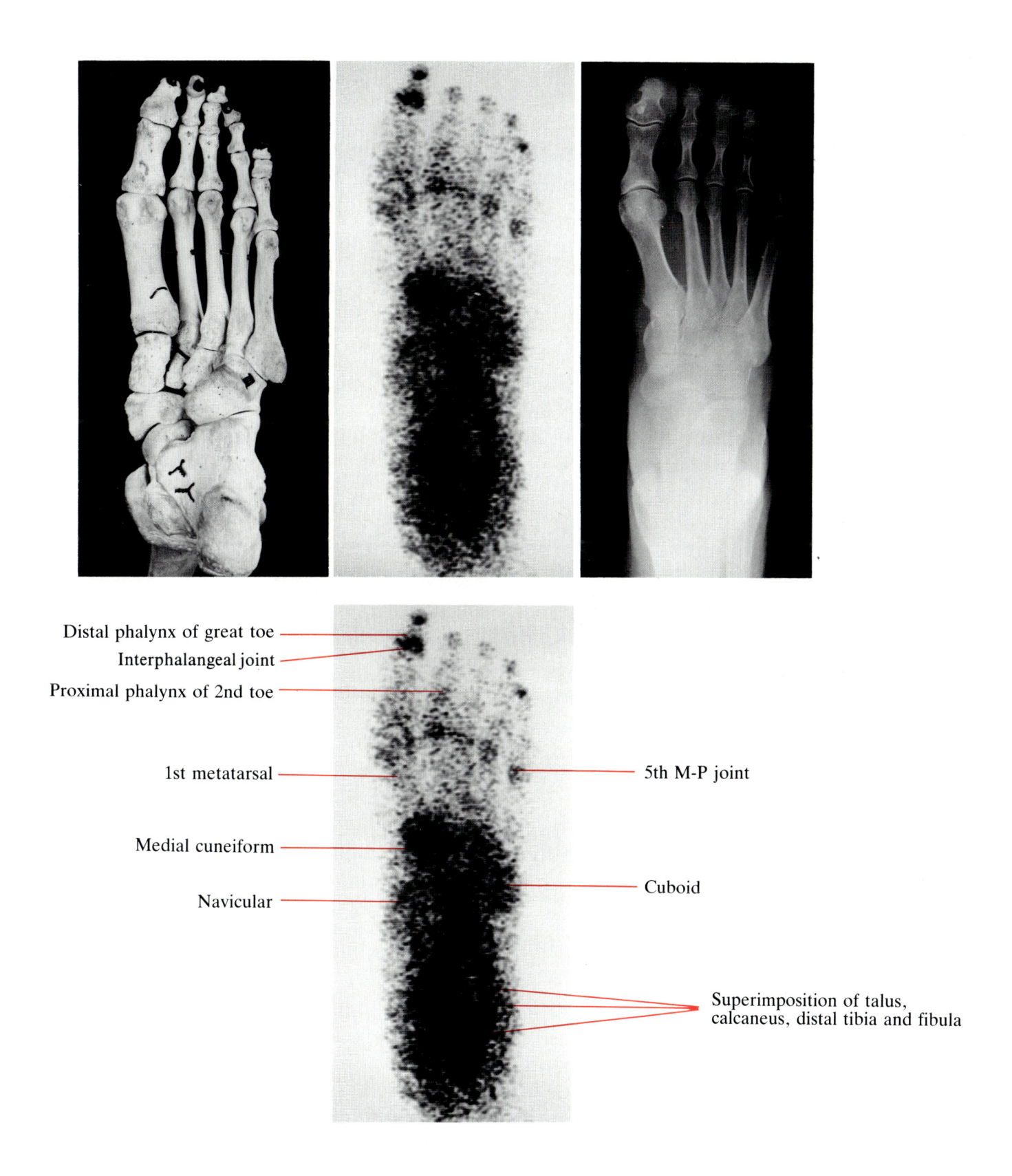

Distal phalynx of great toe
Interphalangeal joint
Proximal phalynx of 2nd toe

1st metatarsal

5th M-P joint

Medial cuneiform

Cuboid

Navicular

Superimposition of talus, calcaneus, distal tibia and fibula